# SUFFICIENT GRACE:
# SURVIVING PROSTATE CANCER

# SUFFICIENT GRACE:
## SURVIVING PROSTATE CANCER

**A Physician Shares His Personal
Spiritual Experience With Prostate Cancer**

**By**

**L. Rudy Broomes, M.D.**

Photographic Credits: The Author

Rudlauv Publishers, LLC
P.O. Box 70893
Tuscaloosa, AL 35407-0893

## FIRST EDITION

Typeset and Printed by University Printing Services
The University of Alabama
Tuscaloosa, AL 35487-0154

*This book is dedicated*
*first, to the memory of my deceased mother, Thelma Morris;*
*to my wife, Lauvenia;*
*to my daughters, Lloyda and Melissa, for their support during my growth*
*and development, professional career, and particularly during the ordeal*
*with the illness about which I write.*
*Second, to all who must function without part(s) of their body.*
*Third, to all who must live with those who function without the part(s).*
*Fourth, to those who make continued functioning possible.*

# ACKNOWLEDGEMENTS

This book has been in the making for a long time. So many people have contributed that I can say emphatically, "It has taken a community to help write it." In my early teens in Trinidad I developed a "way with words." A friend told me that I was good at sarcasm. I was so uninformed that I stood in an uneasy silence and took the statement as a compliment. When I recovered, I mended my ways. During my early years of psychiatric practice I lectured frequently on substance abuse, and on one occasion a social worker in Nashville, Tennessee, asked me if I had written any books. However, over the years, I wrote a number of articles for Message Magazine.

When I finally decided to write I shared my work during a lay preaching engagement. Dr. Timothy Mc Donald of Oakwood College said, upon hearing me, "Rudy, you write from your heart; are you going to publish?" Shortly after that I received the best compliment ever when Pastor T.R. Smith of Atlanta said publicly, "Dr. Broomes, you remind me of an expression we no longer use, 'fellow feel.' You are blessed with the capacity to enable your hearers to feel what you describe." Comments from my family and close friends have been equally inspiring, and for that I am grateful.

I thank all who contributed in making this book a reality. A few people, however, stand out above others. My wife, Lauvenia, was a prime mover every step of the way. She helped not only with the book but also by her brave survival of Lupus for more than twenty-seven years. June Moore challenged my expressions over the telephone on countless occasions and directly. She wanted me to be sure that what I wanted to say was clearly conveyed to the reader who did not have the background information of a close friend. Jeremy Moore highlighted the importance of "dialogue" in writing. My son-in-law, Dennis Williamson, urged me to improve my computer competence by believing in my potential to master the relevant skills and by providing technical assistance here and there.

The objects I made for my self-styled "occupational therapy" are particularly significant for the inspiration I received from my grandchildren, Jonathan and Grace. Instead of going out and purchasing a number of toys and household items, I made them. The knowledge that the children would know that "granddad" made those items was a driving force behind making those items and the recovery about which I write.

Finally, I am deeply indebted to Mrs. Sandra Baldwin for expert advice; Dr. William E. Coopwood for his critical review and the foreword; and Mrs. Shirley Bailey, retired Administrative Assistant and Accreditation Specialist of Oakwood College, Huntsville, Alabama, editor, for their signal contributions.

# FOREWORD

Occasionally life affords us an opportunity to "Stop, Look, and Listen" as it were. We are forced to "Stop" our hectic pace of activities that are deemed by us to be of premier importance at the time. We are challenged to "Look" at an array of introspective options that merit our consideration, and we are provided a "moment" in time to "Listen" to inspirational insights, encouragement, and direction from God.

Dr. Broomes has shared an insightful, extremely honest, and candid rehearsal of his experience with the discovery of his prostate cancer. The reflections on his journeying through his youthful ambivalent search for a significant role for himself in life, the successful focus on a professional career choice as a physician, and the jolting interruption imposed by the discovery of cancer are articulated very clearly in his book. His artful use of a sequence of warm and engaging vignettes vividly depicts his difficult mental, emotional, physical, and spiritual struggles through the ordeal of diagnosis, the dreaded anticipation of surgery, and the painful post-operative phases of his experience.

It is apparent that he has discovered the rich mother lode of treasured spiritual resources that are to be found in Divine Scriptures as evidenced by his ample quoting of relevant Biblical references. He has allowed us to accompany him on this very human journey. He has encouraged us by his sharing with us the soulful remedies that were so effective in facilitating his passage through his "vale of tears." We are grateful for his shared insights, and we are definitely better for them.

William E. Coopwood, M.D.
Medical Director, Senior Services
Deaconess Cross Pointe Hospital
Evansville, Indiana

# PREFACE

The past two years of my life have been eventful ones. From the moment I realized I was diagnosed with prostate cancer that illness took on a whole new meaning. I knew of the illness as a physician and had kept up with the latest aspects via continuing medical education. In fact, a few public figures were reported to have had this condition, about which general information was publicized. Further, of the three of my friends who were similarly diagnosed two had died from it. As the news of my situation spread, I discovered that at least eleven more were in various stages of recovery. Worse yet, I had to invade their privacy to get relevant information.

It was extremely difficult for even friends to share what the experience was like. This was no clinical case conference. It was my life. I now reasoned that God was in charge of my life. He had brought me from a modest upbringing and as an automobile mechanic to several privileged positions and experiences as a psychiatrist. If the time had come for me to die, I would fade away in gratitude. If I should live it meant that I still had a purpose to fulfill. I remembered the words of **Romans 8:28 (NKJV)-"And we know that all things work together for good to those who love God, to those who are called according to His purpose."** And I thought of **2 Corinthians 12:9-"Most gladly therefore will I rather glory in my infirmities."** That purpose was to find the "good" in "all things" and for me to write about the "glory" I found in the lessons I learned from my infirmities. Perhaps I could do something to avoid being a member in the Society of Silent Sufferers. So my reason for this book is to share details of my experience with the diagnosis, treatment, and recovery from prostate cancer, about which men are usually reluctant to speak. The textbooks, pamphlets, and brochures on the subject tell what to expect. I attempt to describe, in part, what it was like for me for the first two years of recovery.

I understand the basis for privacy. After all, urinary incontinence, the loss of the prostate gland, crying in public without warning, insecurity about the future, the loss of procreative ability, etc., are not popular subjects among macho men. Even when such topics come to mind, they are likely to be summarily dismissed. So as I had these experiences, I coupled them with texts of scripture. That's how I survived. That's what I share.

I did not join a specific support group other than to attend church services regularly. However, I made objects in my workshop at my own pace that would be comparable to what I called my "occupational therapy." I particularly liked woodwork although I had only simple tools. As my strength improved I made items of practical use for my family, especially my grandchildren. The dormant hobbies from my youth came in handy now and helped me regain my health. I became more observant about things in my surroundings. River rocks had been everywhere, but I was too busy to notice them until now. I soon discovered that I could convert them into gifts with a personal touch. So I collected, sorted, shellacked, and placed them in a variety of attractive containers.

I had been planning to retire in about two years. However, the turn of events shortened that time to months instead of years. What would I do? How would I spend my time? Working on carpentry and art projects gave me ample opportunities to do a lot of uninterrupted thinking. During this period, poetic and prosaic themes came in torrents. For example, while I was making a toy house from scraps of wood from a broken director's chair I composed an acrostic from MYSTERIES as a metaphor of my life. As I spent more time meditating, planning, and writing, my interest in writing poetry and prose revived. Here I found an ample outlet for self-expression that was not necessarily related to my illness. I survived!

Writing was therapeutic. God promised to heal me, and my medical team could only do so much. I had to do the rest. I identified with how my patients felt–frustrated, unsure, vulnerable, tearful, alone, but hopeful.

# TABLE OF CONTENTS
## PART I: DEVOTIONAL

## COLOR INSERT: SELF-DIRECTED OCCUPATIONAL THERAPY ITEMS

## PART I: CONTINUED

## PART II: POETRY AND PROSE

### PRAYERS

### HOLY SCRIPTURES

### MOTIVATION

### ACROSTICS

### POEMS

### SHORT STORY

# INTRODUCTION

"I am sorry to have to give you this kind of news. But based on my examination and the test results, you have prostate cancer." It does not matter how subdued the doctor tries to sound, that sort of news sounds like a death sentence. "According to the Cleveland Clinic more than 180,000 men in the US would be diagnosed with prostate cancer in 2002, and more than 30,000 would die of the disease". Nevertheless, with the advances in medical care today, neither the announcement nor the statistics have to be as ominous as they sound. Interventions are available to prevent death from this illness if it is detected and treated early enough. This message is the thrust of **Sufficient Grace: Surviving Prostate Cancer**.

One night as I was in the final stages of completing the manuscript for this book the phone rang. The hesitating voice said, "This is Alvin (not his real name). Betsy Jones (not her real name) told me that I could call you." I recognized the names and replied supportively, "Oh, yes, she asked if you could talk to me about your situation. I willingly told her, 'That would be fine with me.' " The caller and I exchanged polite greetings. Then I broke the awkward silence. "I have been expecting to hear from you. I understand that you have a problem that I faced recently." I sensed his characteristic reluctance to talk about prostate issues, so I took the lead in the conversation. After a few minutes, Alvin asked me to talk to his wife who spoke with empathy and professional directness. In a rather short interchange, she covered several critical issues. At the end of the call I paused to reflect on the ease with which three strangers had discussed such a delicate topic. It was then that I realized that I was guided by the sentiments and contents of the three parts of **Sufficient Grace: Surviving Prostate Cancer**.

Part I is a devotional. In it I link sixty-one of the myriad issues I encountered with my diagnosis, treatment, and recovery with texts of scripture. I had dedicated my life to Jesus Christ in my late teens, and He has proven to be a reliable Leader. So now, as a senior citizen, I saw no reason to abandon Him while I dealt with such concerns as shock, uncertainty for the future, surgery, possible death, recovery, friends, family, healing, etc. Further, I was convinced that the Scriptures contained realistic aid for these challenging circumstances. I kept the accounts brief on purpose. I did not want the information to overwhelm the reader who might be fearful of what lay ahead, particularly at a time of feeling vulnerable. At the same time larger sections could be covered, if desired.

The Color Insert Section emphasizes the importance of staying as busy as can be tolerated. Woodworking is one of my hobbies. So I made items for practical use by my family who were supportive of my activities. In fact, one item, the kiddies canvas bookshelf, is a joint project. The idea was suggested by one of my daughters, I made the frame, and my wife sewed the one-piece canvas shelf. Another piece, the oak trunk plant stand, is my wife's brainchild. She spotted a stump of wood among some recently discarded logs at a construction site and mentioned that

I might be able to do something with it. I did. The river rock collection seemed silly at first. However, as I washed and polished the stones, and placed them in attractive glass or plastic containers, their hidden beauty emerged. I took time to interact with the natural environment around me.

The Poetry and Prose in Part II provide yet another fruitful outlet since my thoughts and feelings included concerns beyond my illness. I used the poetic format of acrostics to express how I dealt with issues like acceptance, disability, frustration, and recovery. However, life situations like relationships, nature, recreation, stress, and the importance of the Holy Scriptures crossed my mind with intense impressions that I felt I had to record. For example, I had seen parodies on the Twenty-third Psalm dealing with the addict, the alcoholic, and the television. So I yielded to the urge to compose the Psalm of the Prostate. Finally, in this section, I place original eponyms as fillers between the poetic items. The expressions enclosed in brackets in some of these statements are usually thought of but not expressed out loud.

Current medical literature now regularly includes the psychological components of the reaction to medical/surgical illness. Recently, however, the positive spiritual influence on recovery from illness is being included with increasing frequency. The accounts include research findings as well as anecdotal reports. **Sufficient Grace: Surviving Prostate Cancer** is a description of how spirituality helped me to cope with my illness during the two most challenging years of my life.

# PART I: DEVOTIONAL

## SILENCE

The moment I learned of my diagnosis over the phone I shrank into silence. In my earlier years, I was a shy person. As I grew older that changed – particularly after completing my training as a psychiatrist. I enjoyed lecturing on Substance Dependence and other mental health subjects, and conducting seminars on Family Relations with my wife. Now it appeared that I was about to return to my former style. I was at work and for a few moments I could not function. Fortunately, I had no patients in my office at the time. I collected my thoughts sufficiently to let my supervisor know that I had just received some disturbing news about my health, and that I was in no condition to treat patients. However, I would finish the morning schedule.

My wife and I were expecting to hear from the doctor's office. But when I showed up at home at noon with my attaché case, untouched lunch bag, flushed face, dazed eyes, and tightly blanched lips my body language said it all. We hugged at the door! Time stood still! Finally I said, "I have cancer." The news meant that benign prostatic hyperplasia with atypical cells – the previous diagnosis – deteriorated into adenocarcinoma of the prostate. I wasn't reading this statement from a patient's chart. I wasn't reading an article in a medical journal. I wasn't attending a noon surgical conference that was scheduled between ward rounds and office visits with a brown-bag lunch provided by a pharmaceutical company. Malignant cells were rapidly multiplying in my body – wherever the blood vessels or lymph channels would take them. When I revived, I looked beyond myself. I looked to God for direction. We looked to God for direction.

**"Be still and know that I am God" (Psalm 46:10).**

———— ◆ ————

## HURT

When we are ignored, we hurt. When life does not seem fair, we hurt. When my mother whipped me and called out my catalogued childhood infractions with each stroke of a leather belt, I hurt. When I fell through the kitchen floor of my childhood home, the protruding nail dug into my right leg. At first the flesh seemed pale before the blood oozed out. I was afraid; and I was hurt, too. That was more than sixty years ago. The scene, however, is still very fresh in my mind. Some hurts just don't go away. The intensity may vary and the memory may not be as clear. But something persists. Sometimes the hurt returns and you can see it coming. On other occasions, however, some unsuspecting trigger allows an instant recall of the original experience, causing a reaction that is out of proportion to the matter at hand to interrupt an otherwise calm conversation. That's what happened to me.

Now I waited to be scheduled for surgery, and I started to hurt again. Would I feel any pain? What if the anesthesia wore off too quickly? What if the pain medication was not strong enough? What if the nurse was too busy with another patient and delayed with my pill? After all, I had cancer, but I felt no physical pain. I conjured up a long list of "what ifs." So this is what it is like to have cancer. Me? Cancer? Again, I sought the Lord for relief and direction.

**"They shall not hurt nor destroy in all my holy mountain: for the earth shall be full of the knowledge of the Lord, as the waters cover the sea" (Isaiah 11:9).**

---

## SHOCK

In medicine, there are four basic kinds of shock: first, a condition in which the cells of the body receive inadequate amounts of oxygen due to changes in perfusion; second, a sudden physical or biochemical disturbance that results in inadequate blood flow to vital organs; third, a state of profound mental and physical depression that is the result of severe physical injury or an emotional disturbance; fourth, a state characterized by inadequacy of blood flow throughout the body to the extent that damage occurs to the cells of the tissues. In addition, *The PDR Medical Dictionary*, Second Edition, p. 1631, Medical Economics Company, 2000 Lippincott Williams and Wilkins lists over thirty different types of shock.

When the impact of my condition dawned on me, I was in shock: the third kind listed above. Issues of uncertainty, complications, disfigurement, depression, anxiety, and sadness flipped through my mind in rapid succession. I felt myself losing control of my emotions at work. I had patients to attend to and their condition had to take priority over any catastrophe I was experiencing. However, I was in no condition to be responsible for the lives and welfare of other people. I prayed to God. I had critical decisions to make in the next few minutes.

**"When you pass through the waters, I will be with you" (Isaiah 43:2, NKJV).**

## PAST

As human beings, we are very fortunate that we are not continually aware of all our past experiences. We would be quite miserable if these memories were not unconsciously stored for future reference, as needed. However, there are times when the past is summoned into the present whether you want it or not. Triggers have a way of doing just that. The word "adenocarcinoma" meant malignant cancer. It was a powerful trigger; it forced me to review my life:

Scenes of my modest upbringing as a boy in Trinidad, West Indies,

Scenes of my early occupation as an automobile mechanic with Shell Oil Company,

Scenes of my professional development in medical school,

Scenes of prior surgery for tonsillectomy and carpal tunnel syndrome,

Scenes of the fate of men who had a similar diagnosis, and many more passed before my mind's eyes. What a vivid mental videotape I reviewed! I did some serious thinking about my relationship with God over and beyond my usual meditations. Did my past experiences count for anything?

**"Oh, that I were as in months past, As in the days when God watched over me; When His lamp shone upon my head, And when by His light I walked through darkness; Just as I was in the days of my prime, When the friendly counsel of God was over my tent" (Job 29:2-4, NKJV).**

## PRESENT

We were in the midst of a psychotherapy session when a patient told me that she was confused. "That's good," I said with a smile. She did not think that was amusing, and she told me so. I stated that it was not my intent to belittle her. I then explained to her that it was to her advantage to realize that she was confused. Our task now was to identify the various aspects of her confusion so she could be relieved of her distress. She pondered my response and continued cautiously. She agreed to explore private areas of her confused life.

Like her, I realized I was dealing with several apparently conflicting thoughts and emotions. I thought I understood God, but now He was not making sense. Bad things were happening to me, a good person. I followed a healthy diet, now look at what happened! I had become accustomed to telling my patients and friends who sought my counsel that in order to "get over" something there are times when you have to "go through" it. Now it was my turn to reach out to God and to those who could bring relief.

**"And it shall come to pass, that before they call, I will answer; and while they are yet speaking, I will hear" (Isaiah 65:24).**

## FUTURE

A long time ago I heard someone say that today is the tomorrow we worried about yesterday. I lead a busy life. From my childhood I had been programmed to fill every minute with sixty seconds of useful activities. It made sense. My wife had been encouraging me to slow down for some time. When I did not ignore her I responded with angry rationalizations. She reminded me from time to time of the numerous stories of family, friends, and strangers who could not enjoy their retirement because they had lived at too fast a pace. In some instances, some of them even died before retirement. I made up excuses. I flashed ambitious plans before her. After all, we wanted to travel; we wanted to pay off the mortgage ahead of time; we had to plan for comfortable sunset years. In fact, my anticipated retirement date was not very far away. We were actually counting down. I was even supposed to write a book. I had learned all the usual male "you-have-to-be-productive-and-show-it" values.

Now, as I pondered the future, I wondered whether any of those plans really mattered.

**"Do not be overly righteous, Nor be overly wise: Why would you destroy yourself? (Ecclesiastes 7:16, NKJV)**

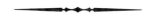

## ALONE

Experience cannot be obtained through proxy. It does not matter how many good wishes come your way. It does not matter what kind of instructions you receive. It does not matter if someone wished they could be a substitute for you. Some things you have to do for yourself. I was scheduled for surgery, and I was the one who would undergo the procedure. That did not mean, however, that I was not going to be in a very supportive environment. In order to provide an environment of inclusiveness for singles and the challenges they faced, the motto YANA was developed: You Are Not Alone. Although sin has brought miseries of all kinds, diseases of various degrees of devastation, and the resulting death, we do not have to suffer in a state of aloneness.

As I faced the process of diagnosis, treatment, and recovery, the experience was mine. The medical team was competent; my family was supportive; my church reminded me of hope that is available in times like these. But the experience was mine alone.

Jesus felt the burden of our sins in the Garden of Gethsemane and looked to His disciples for support. They failed Him, so He called upon His Father. Ben H. Price, in the hymn, *Alone,* said of Jesus, "Forsaken then by God and man. Alone, His life He gave." Rodeheaver's Gospel Solos and Duets, No. 1. (47) Jesus showed us how to handle aloneness. In Christ we may be alone, but never lonely.

**"I will not leave you nor forsake you" (Joshua 1:5, NKJV).**

## SUPPORT

The title of the last sermon I preached before my surgery was, "The Society of Silent Sufferers and their Circle of Support." When the word got out that I had cancer, a number of fellow believers shared only tidbits of their silent woes. "How tragic!" I thought. Many could not speak freely, even in private settings. In fact, it appeared that the degree of reluctance to talk about illnesses was not related to level of education or severity of the condition. Some were close friends. They were perhaps as frightened and as vulnerable as I was. Frequently the conversation switched to trading passages of scripture. Sharing concerns on a feeling level was rare, and its lack accentuated my disappointment and quandary. No wonder we appear so gloomy in church services. Many burdened people feel crushed and simply stay away from the fellowship of believers.

By mentioning my plight in public, I was getting some relief, but I was ignoring the Code of the Silent Sufferers: "Don't say anything." I appealed to the congregation at the end of my discourse and invited all who were suffering in one way or the other to join me in the aisle in front of the pulpit. Then I encouraged those people who had not responded thus far to form a Circle of Support around us. Many who were reluctant to talk about their aches, pains, and miseries readily responded to the altar call.

I was happy and gratified for the demonstration of caring and support we gave to each other.

**"Bear one another's burdens" (Galatians 6:2, NKJV).**

------◆◆◆------

## FRIENDS

My family moved several times while I was growing up. Some of the changes I liked and others I did not. So making lasting friendships was very tenuous for me. Before I was married, I had moved ten times. No, I did not belong to a Uniformed Services family. Looking back, I think we were just trying to rise above the poverty zone. Then by the time of my illness my wife and I had been married for thirty-seven years. In that period we had relocated fifteen times: blame it on medical school and psychiatry residency training and medical practice opportunities. As word of my condition spread we heard from friends from all over the United States and overseas. This gesture was very comforting. It went a long way to balance my sense of isolation. We were out of sight for varying periods of time and from numerous locations, but we were not out of mind.

The concern warmed our hearts. It made me think that's what God is like. We cannot see Him, but we know He is there.

**"A man who has friends must himself be friendly, But there is a friend who sticks closer than a brother" (Proverbs 18:24, NKJV).**

------◆◆◆------

## FAMILY

My desire to realize my ambition to become a physician meant that I had to migrate to the United States of America. Ten years passed before my first return to Trinidad to visit my family. Since then I made trips every four to five years; but the closeness was never the same. We all changed. Respect and awe replaced familiarity. I missed them when I was away and felt awkward when I visited. New generations were born, and in-laws joined our family.

When I learned of the severity of my illness, I phoned and wrote letters to describe my condition. The silence that followed confirmed my suspicions. The price of distance and time from relatives was evident. At least, so I thought. My surgery came and went. I did not hear anything from my family. Did they not care what happened to me? At least, if they cared, could they not show it? Then after what appeared to be an eternity and exaggerated short-term effects of general anesthesia, the phone in my hospital room rang.

My wife took the call and said it was from my nephew. She gave me the phone. Suddenly I mattered! He cared! He knew the surgery schedule and wanted a progress report from me personally. So he waited long enough for me to regain my strength in order to contact me directly for details. When I got off the phone I cried for joy. He promised to relay the report to the other family members, and that was good enough for me.

There are times when we have to allow the people around us to love us in their own way and on their own schedule. They have their reasons for doing things their way: just like we have our reasons, too. I learned to accept their love and concern on their terms.

**"For now I see in a mirror, dimly, but then face to face. Now I know in part, but then I shall just as I also am known. And now abide faith, hope, love, these three; but the greatest of these is love" (1 Corinthians 13:12, 13, NKJV).**

## COLLEAGUES

I wondered about my colleagues. What were they thinking of me? What were they saying? Would I ever be able to rejoin their ranks? Would their conversation about male reproductive body parts change in my presence? Would they see me simply as data in cancer statistics? As for colleagues with a religious background I had my concerns, too. One friend stated that I looked too healthy to have cancer. Another one proclaimed that he hoped that the surgeon would not find any cancer when he did the surgery. No one, in my case: however, inquired out loud if the calamity was punishment for some sin committed by one of my predecessors or by me. After all, it crossed my mind. But one thing was clear: My colleagues were genuinely concerned about me and they came to be supportive.

On one occasion I felt sufficiently comfortable to tell a small group what was on my heart. I had surrendered my life to God a long time ago; He had blessed me beyond my wildest dreams; and now benign prostatic hyperplasia had changed to adenocarcinoma. I sought the best care available locally. If the Lord would not allow me to survive the illness, I was satisfied with Him; but if I lived, then perhaps my purpose in life was not fully realized. Praises be to God! I am convinced that telling my story is part of that purpose.

**"Being confident of this very thing, that he which hath begun a good work in you will perform it until the day of Jesus Christ" (Philippians 1:6).**

— ◆ —

## STRANGERS

A few weeks into my recovery, I ventured into a grocery store with my wife to assist with the shopping. I was so preoccupied with my plight, it seemed as though every one I saw knew about my illness. My gait was slow and deliberate; my posture was erect. Pushing the grocery cart provided for a good camouflage. That way, the cart became the center of attention–except that it was empty for a while. My mental condition accentuated what little physical discomfort I was experiencing. Suddenly I felt tearful. I excused myself immediately and went to the car in the parking lot. It did not matter that my thoughts were irrational. It did not matter that shoppers were too engrossed in their own affairs–wearing the latest fads and looking for the best unit price. It did not matter that my wife needed my help with the grocery cart while she actually did the shopping. I had to leave the scene. The self-consciousness was overwhelming.

The expectations I had of strangers without their knowledge or consent was a powerful stimulus. It made me behave in an uncharacteristic manner. That's what my mind-set did to me.

However, when we know God and His will for us we can face any mishap successfully. The anguish of illness became a fleeting experience although I felt it from time to time with decreasing frequency and intensity.

**"How precious also are thy thoughts unto me, O God! How great is the sum of them!" (Psalms 139:17).**

## RELIEF

Some cancers occur in one place at the primary or main location. Others may invade the tissues that surround the particular organ. That's bad enough. But perhaps the most ominous condition is the presence of cancer cells in multiple places beyond the original location: beyond the primary site. In other words, some cancers metastasize. When I was sufficiently awake in the recovery room my urologist told me that he had successfully removed my prostate and in the process he had also examined several of my pelvic lymph nodes. They appeared normal. However, it would be a few days before he could relay a conclusive report from the pathologist.

Two days passed, then the phone rang. I recognized my doctor's voice; for I had grown to know him well over the time he had been treating me. He said, "I have good news for you. The cancer was confined to the prostate. It did not even involve the capsule tissue. Best of all, the pathologist said that all the lymph nodes are clear." He continued, "You are cured." That was indeed providential news. I received another miracle. Needless to say, I cried for joy right there in my hospital bed. I felt relieved. There were no cancer cells growing out of control in my body!

When I was in my late teens, I delayed completing my decision for Christ by postponing my baptism. I agonized for four years about that decision. Then the day came when I finally fulfilled my promise to God and was baptized into the fellowship of Christians. What a relief that was, too!

It is comforting to know that Jesus removed the uncertainty of an aimless life and an unknown future by His invitation to take Him at His word. We do not have to be anxious about problems He has already solved. In spite of the vicissitudes in our lives the outcome can be certain.

**"Come now, and let us reason together, saith the LORD: though your sins be as scarlet, they shall be as white as snow; though they be red like crimson, they shall be as wool" (Isaiah 1:18).**

# HEALING

Ambroise Paré, the French surgeon, once said that it was his responsibility to dress wounds, and it was God who did the healing. My previous surgeries went well. I healed on schedule. I wondered if this experience might be different because the diagnosis was more ominous and the operation more complicated. I remembered a statement that surgeons allegedly make at heroic surgical feats with disappointing results: "The operation was a success, but the patient died." Now that my life was at stake, the joke was no longer funny.

During a church service, I asked for support for the ordeal I faced. It came quickly and in different forms. A member of my church pulled me aside.
She gave me a list of eight Bible texts.
She instructed me to study the verses faithfully.
She told me to claim the healing.
She knew the Power of those texts of scripture.
She spoke with confidence.
I scribbled down the texts as she quoted them.
I wrote out the verses and studied them.
I claimed the healing.
I received the Power promised in the passages.
Now I speak with confidence.
It worked!

**"Surely he hath borne our griefs, and carried our sorrows: yet we did esteem him stricken, smitten of God, and afflicted. But he was wounded for our transgressions, he was bruised for our iniquities: the chastisement of our peace was upon him; and with his stripes we are healed" (Isaiah 53:4, 5).**

# DOLDRUMS

I must have been in an elementary school nature study class when I was taught about the weather condition called doldrums. In oceanic areas close to the equator there are periods of dead calm and light fluctuating winds. Ships that depend on the wind for travel do not make much progress under these conditions.

So it was with me. There were times during my recovery when I did not know whether I was going or coming. I kept my doctor's appointments, took the medications as they were prescribed, did the bladder neck exercises faithfully, and tried to be as active as my strength allowed. I concocted vague measurements of progress that did not hold up. But that did not mean that the healing process was not continuing and that God was not watching over me.

**"But now thus saith the LORD that created thee, O Jacob, and he that formed thee, O Israel, Fear not: for I have redeemed thee, I have called thee by thy name; thou art mine. When thou passest through the waters, I will be with thee; and through the rivers, they shall not overflow thee: when thou walkest through the fire, thou shalt not be burned; neither shall the flame kindle upon thee. For I am the LORD thy God, the Holy One of Israel, thy Saviour: I gave Egypt for thy ransom, Ethiopia and Seba for thee" (Isaiah 43:1-3).**

---

## HOPE

Hope was a powerful motivator. It defied the odds. It propelled me to keep moving toward recovery. I remember quite clearly asking silent questions like, "What's going to happen to me?" and "Will I ever be my old self again?" I kept those concerns to myself since I was fully aware that no one had satisfactory answers. I could not share with them all of the factors that went into my questions. To do that would only expose me as a weak, doubting person. So as compassionate as the people around me were, they would not be able to grasp the intensity of my concerns.

The thought often crossed my mind that Christians frequently took their burdens to Christ while they were praying and they picked them back up when they finished. I decided to hope for the best and to direct my energies toward my healing process. After all, I had done my ABCs (Asked, Believed, Claimed). That is what I had become accustomed to telling other people.

**"Come unto Me, all you who labor and are heavy laden, and I will give you rest" (Matthew 11:28, NKJV).**

## PURPOSE

One of the most frequently asked questions when calamities occur is, "Why did this or that happen to me?" At some point in my several years as a psychiatrist I encouraged patients to replace that question with a different one: "What can I learn from this or that?" The first question encourages theories and suppositions, while the second one leads to practical and useful discoveries.

Now it was my turn. I had ample opportunity to examine and apply all the advice I had dished out over the years. Fortunately, I usually practiced what I recommended. Now that the questions were mine, it was I who wanted answers. I needed to see the purpose in my predicament, and I found it. It was now my opportunity for the pages of my experience to document another chapter in the drama of my life. That satisfied me. I had done a lot of talking. It was now time for demonstration.

**"We are hard pressed on every side, yet not crushed; we are perplexed, but not in despair; persecuted, but not forsaken; struck down, but not destroyed–always carrying about in the body the dying of the Lord Jesus, that the life of Jesus also may also be manifested in our body" (2 Corinthians 4: 8-10, NKJV).**

## TESTS

One thing was certain: there were lots of tests. My annual employee checkup included a physical examination, an electrocardiogram, chest x-rays, and tests on my body fluids. I also reported to my family physician. He repeated some of the tests so that he could assess the need for further investigations. When my family physician referred me to the urologist he had his own routine so he could confirm or clarify the seriousness of my condition. We did not take the diagnosis of adenocarcinoma of the prostate lightly. When the urologist scheduled me for surgery I went to the hospital for additional tests in preparation for the operation. And, of course, more tests were done while I was in the hospital in order to monitor my postoperative status. Upon my discharge from the hospital, tests were scheduled at follow-up office visits.

The medical teams had to be sure not only that my diagnosis was correct, but also that I was physically fit to survive the operation. Once I was discharged, my condition was monitored as well. Nothing was left to chance in order to avoid a prolonged convalescence.

God created us. Then He redeemed us. Now He is preparing us to live with Him in the New Earth. But while we are here we must be tested and tried to see if we can be trusted with that gracious gift.

**"What do you conspire against the Lord?  He will make an utter end of it. Affliction will not rise up a second time" (Nahum 1:9, NKJV).**

———◆◆◆———

BIOPSY

The urologist to whom I was referred agreed that although my PSA (Prostate Specific Antigen) was not high, a one hundred percent increase was sufficient justification for a biopsy and an ultrasound test to be done. A biopsy. Nothing to it! I thought. I'd had one done on another occasion: just a routine precaution for reassurance that nothing unusual was going on. The procedure was scheduled, and I showed up with confidence. All that had to be done consisted essentially of allowing samples of my prostate gland to be removed and sent to a pathologist for examination. Microscopic pieces of the tissue would be stained and placed on a glass slide. The trained eye of the specialist would compare what was seen with accepted standard samples, and a verdict would be given. That was straightforward. The previous biopsy was not painful, but the second one was. At any rate the discomfort was fleeting.

What would our spiritual experience be like if we responded to God in that manner? There are several instances in the Scriptures where we are invited to test God that way. Here is my favorite example:

**"Test all things; hold fast what is good" (1Thessalonians 5:21, NKJV).**

———◆◆◆———

# RESULTS

At the end of the visit for the biopsy my urologist indicated that an appointment would be necessary to discuss the results he expected to receive from the pathologist. When I showed up for the appointment he invited me to his office, not the examining room, and urged my wife to join us. We complied. I glanced at his desk. I surveyed his certificates and paintings of southern sceneries. I looked at anatomical models of body parts pertinent to a urologist. The decor was one of order, competence, and relaxation. I was curious and anxious. But this was not the time for interior decoration. Neither was it the time to assess his credentials. I had already done that when my family doctor made the referral.

The sound of shuffling papers in his hand brought me back to reality. He had the blood tests report, the ultrasound pictures, and the biopsy opinion. It was time to tell us the results. Indeed, the PSA was not unusually high, but the change was significant; the ultrasound showed one area of abnormal activity; the biopsy revealed malignant cells in one of the six samples. He told us that the cancer was growing at a moderate rate, about a Gleason Grade 6. In lay language, the condition was not an emergency but it required prompt attention. My wife and I asked a few questions, but he affirmed that the test results were conclusive. Urinary hesitation! No pain! Malignant cancer! Moderate growth rate! Localized? What next?

On one occasion Jesus gave Peter, James, and John some test results about their condition. They had not asked Jesus for His opinion, but due to the seriousness of their state, and in spite of His "sorrowfulness unto death," He paused long enough to tell them what He thought. They had the results and the rest was up to them.

**"And he cometh unto the disciples, and findeth them asleep, and saith unto Peter, What, could ye not watch with me one hour? Watch and pray, that ye enter not into temptation: the spirit indeed is willing, but the flesh is weak "** **(Matthew 26: 40, 41).**

---

## TELEPHONE PRAYER

One of my goddaughters, Zania, upon hearing of my ordeal, phoned to talk to me. Characteristic of my style to control situations and partially denying the seriousness of my illness, I asked about her plans to further her education and learned that she was in the process of enrolling in medical school. She updated me on her latest plans and politely interjected that the call was for me and wondered how I was handling the illness and impending surgery. She took charge of the conversation. I was touched by her maturity and did my best to compose myself. We chatted for a while, and then she said, "Uncle Rudy, would you mind if I prayed for you right now?" I acquiesced readily. Again, I tried to conceal my misty eyes and hesitant speech. My little girl had grown up.

When we hung up I got the distinct impression that my healing was already under way. She was the latest angel God sent to minister to me.

**"Let no man despise thy youth; but be thou an example of the believers, in word, in conversation, in charity, in spirit, in faith, in purity" (1 Timothy 4:12).**

## IGNORANCE

There were gaps in my knowledge base of prostate cancer. Although I was aware of enough concepts to keep up with basic medical education, many years had passed since I had attended classes in anatomy, physiology, neurology, pathology, human sexual response, and subjects related to the function of the prostate gland. I was not completely ignorant. However, I was not sufficiently conversant with the subject to my own satisfaction. What little I remembered did not satisfy me.

So I did what my wife did when she had to educate herself about Lupus. She went on a reading campaign. Now it was my turn. I even bravely picked up brochures on the racks in my doctor's office in addition to the reading material he gave me. (You know what it is like when you are in public and you want to pick up an item without drawing attention to yourself.) I did not read in order to counsel a patient. I read to re-educate myself – to reduce my level of ignorance and the accompanying anxiety. Fortunately, I had access to an abundance of reference material from pamphlets, medical journals, and textbooks. I knew about the subject, but I did not know the subject thoroughly. And that lack of knowledge made me feel uncertain, vulnerable, and anxious.

On many occasions the Apostle Paul specifically addressed the knowledge base of his converts in a direct manner. On one such episode he was dealing with attitudes toward departed loved ones. Seeing the gaps of information and how they lead to false conclusions, Paul had to intervene.

**"But I do not want you to be ignorant, brethren, concerning those who have fallen asleep, lest you sorrow as others who have no hope" (1 Thessalonians 4:13, NKJV).**

## OPTIONS

With the diagnosis now confirmed, and the rate of growth of the cancer established, it was now time for me to decide what to do, when to do it, and where. Observation and monitoring (watchful care), as a treatment option, had already been done. And since it did not appear that the cancer had spread, radiation therapy was one option. However, given my family circumstances, the most appropriate option seemed to be a radical prostatectomy. My doctor stated that I was entitled to a second opinion and that we should call him about our final decision.

But my wife and I had already anticipated what he would say.

We had already prayed to God for guidance.

We had read the medical references on prostate cancer treatment the doctor gave us.

We had talked to a few close friends.

We had talked to a number of prostate cancer survivors.

We had asked our church family to pray also.

Without hesitation we gave the doctor our decision:

"Schedule the operation as soon as possible."


**"Where no counsel is, the people fall: but in the multitude of counselors there is safety" (Proverbs 11:14).**


## BLOOD

I donated two pints of blood to myself, as advised, prior to surgery just in case I need it: autologous transfusions. Perhaps there are two issues that make such transfusions necessary. First, it avoids the transmission of unsuspecting illnesses from one person to another. Second, most blood banks have a short supply. Although considerable blood loss was not expected, the surgeon was preparing for a possible emergency.

Great care had to be taken to ensure the integrity of the transfusion process. Sterility, storage conditions, identification systems, preservation, and double-checking with another qualified staff member are among the precautions that are observed with the strictest professionalism. Any deviation could have led to unnecessary or tragic consequences when the blood was reintroduced into my circulatory system.

The introduction of sin into this world resulted in the shedding of Christ's blood on the cross to bring about our redemption. It is only as we accept that sacrifice that we are counted worthy of salvation. Otherwise we are lost. God has set up the conditions for reconciliation that we must follow explicitly.

**"And almost all things are by the law purged with blood; and without shedding of blood is no remission. It was therefore necessary that the patterns of things in the heavens should be purified with these; but the heavenly things themselves with better sacrifices than these" (Hebrews 9:22, 23).**

---

## SURGERY

I decided to have the surgery done in a local hospital. Friends suggested that I should go out of town to one of two nationally famous medical centers. I realized that an out-of-town location would give me access to excellent medical care. However, it would deprive me of the necessary family support for a sustained period of time, and that family members would have to make several stressful trips to be with me. Given our family situation, even remaining local was demanding on them.

I reasoned that God had shaped circumstances to allow the cancer to be detected in its early stage; He had directed me to the best possible choice of an option; He had the power to perform whatever kind of miracle He deemed appropriate; and that since He could heal me at a distant location, He could heal me locally. God's power is not limited by geography.

**"Then Jesus went with them. And when he was now not far from the house, the centurion sent friends to him, saying unto him, Lord, trouble not thyself: for I am not worthy that thou shouldest enter under my roof: Wherefore neither thought I myself worthy to come unto thee: but say in a word, and my servant shall be healed" (Luke 7: 6, 7).**

## SURRENDER

I experienced a vivid example of surrendering on the night of my first postoperative day when my family lovingly decided to take turns sitting with me. That night, I felt the urge to use the toilet and groaned, "I want to go to the bathroom." My older daughter, a physician, was by herself. She tried to reassure me by declaring, "Dad, you have a Foley catheter." "I want to use the toilet!" I mumbled, in order to indicate that she did not understand the urgency of my announcement. In my state of mind, it did not matter that there was nothing substantial in my lower bowel that required a trip to the bathroom. So, I held on to the side rail indicating by my body language that I was about to go to the toilet a few blurry feet away: never mind the I.V. line; never mind the Foley catheter; never mind my immediate post-anesthetic condition. I remember her saying emphatically, "Dad, you're not getting up." (Or was it her body language?) I completely relaxed.

I surrendered. I gave in. I didn't say another word. She was in charge and we both knew it. There comes a time in our relationship with the Lord when that is the only sensible thing to do: Surrender unconditionally.

**"Then he fell to the ground, and heard a voice saying to him, 'Saul, Saul, why are you persecuting Me?" And he said, 'Who are You, Lord?' Then the Lord said, 'I am Jesus, whom you are persecuting. It is hard for you to kick against the goads.' So he, trembling and astonished, said, 'Lord, what do You want me to do?' Then the Lord said to him, 'Arise and go into the city, and you will be told what you must do'"** (Acts 9:4-6, NKJV).

## CATHETER

The surgical procedure I underwent involved my urethra, the natural conduit that provides for the passage of the urine collected in my bladder to flow to the outside. The waste fluid could not be allowed to remain in my bladder or to flow freely into my abdominal cavity for any appreciable length of time. Until that part of the urethra healed, I was fitted with a Foley catheter. It does not slip out because of the retaining balloon at the end that extends into the urinary bladder. The other end is attached to plastic bag for collection and measurement of urine output. This substitute tube is a critical item that contributes immensely to the success of the surgery. Even when the cancer is completely removed, the tissues at the surgical site must be protected from conditions that would undermine the healing process. Thus, a substitute must be provided.

That's what Jesus did for us. We were estranged from God when Adam and Eve sinned. None of us could satisfy the value of the ransom, so He paid the redemptive penalty. He died in our place. He became the Perfect Substitute to reconcile us to God.

**"And I will put enmity between thee and the woman, and between thy seed and her seed; it shall bruise thy head, and thou shalt bruise his heel" (Genesis 3:15).**

---

## RECOVERY

I was intensely concerned about my ability to get back on my feet. I wondered how I would adapt without a prostate.

Would my tissues heal on schedule?

When would I resume regular activities?

How about my stamina?

How would I also continue to adjust to being a senior citizen?

What if I developed complications?

Would I experience medication side effects?

What would happen if I had an emergency?

Would I ever be able to keep up with work pressures?

During my many years of delivering patient care, I had guided hundreds of patients through their recuperation. I used to tell them that "the only way out of a situation" was to "go through it." Now the tables were turned. Although I had had major surgery before, I wondered if my recovery on this occasion was going to be different.

**"But they that wait upon the LORD shall renew their strength; they shall mount up with wings as eagles; they shall run, and not be weary; and they shall walk, and not faint" (Isaiah 40:31).**

## INSTRUCTIONS

My doctor stated that he would discharge me from the hospital when he thought I was sufficiently stable. He finally wrote the discharge order, but I could not leave until the nurses and other members of the staff gave me the prescribed instructions. Those words reminded me of the discharge process I used with my patients. How closely would I follow these instructions, I wondered. After all, my patients occasionally wanted me to hasten the formality and listened to me out of respect. Some of them cared little about what I had to say. And in the discharge summary I had to indicate whether or not the patient or some other responsible person understood what I had explained to them. Were discharge instructions an important factor in recovery? Now it was my turn to find out.

The seriousness of my illness and the delicacy of the surgery were made clear. I had to limit strenuous activity until my doctor authorized it. I had prescriptions to fill and follow-up appointments to keep. The consequences were explained and the results were up to me.

**"See, I have set before thee this day life and good, and death and evil; In that I command thee this day to love the LORD thy God, to walk in his ways, and to keep his commandments and his statutes and his judgments, that thou mayest live and multiply: and the LORD thy God shall bless thee in the land whither thou goest to possess it. But if thine heart turn away, so that thou wilt not hear, but shalt be drawn away, and worship other gods, and serve them; I denounce unto you this day, that ye shall surely perish, and that ye shall not prolong your days upon the land, whither thou passest over Jordan to go to possess it" (Deuteronomy 30:15-18).**

## PRAYER

I composed a seven-point prayer several years ago and had a habit of sharing it in Relationship Seminars that my wife and I conducted. Now I needed those seven points in a focused manner for myself. In an abbreviated form it states: 1. Father, help me to know Your will for my life. 2. Please bring to my attention whatever I need in order to meet the challenges of relating to others and to get ready for Jesus' coming. 3. Please do not let what You reveal scare me. 4. If I cannot handle by myself what You show me, please send some assistance and help me to recognize it. 5. Please help to get it right early and not to have to go through the turmoil to change too many times. 6. Help me to remember that others are struggling, too. 7. Father, thank You for Your concern.

Somehow I had the impression that the things I had been doing in my life thus far were preparing me to handle the present challenges. No wonder it has been said that the past is prologue.

**"O thou that hearest prayer, unto thee shall all flesh come" (Psalms 65:2).**

———◆———

## SCRIPTURES

There were many days when I did not want to read. I did not even want to look at the colorful pictures in books–one of my favorite carry-overs from childhood. Watching television was even less enticing. The Lord knew what I needed, though, and how to supply it. It was at those times that Scriptures I learned in my formative years popped into my waiting mind.

Not only that: in many cases, the circumstances under which I learned those precious memory verses returned quite vividly. How comforting! How appropriate! In those early years of important growth and development my mother, church members like Mr. Medford Francis, and surrogate parents like Mrs. Leontine Mitchell insisted that I memorize passages of Scripture. Often, against childhood protests, in a foggy state of mind for mandatory family morning worship, I stored away the words. Now, in my sunset years, the messages of encouragement and hope came to fulfill their divine mission, as if programmed to do so.

**"And these words which I command you today shall be in your heart; You shall teach them diligently to your children, and shall talk of them when you sit in your house, when you walk by the way, when you lie down, and when you rise up" (Deuteronomy 6:6, 7, NKJV).**

## BELIEFS

My illness tested my beliefs. All of the things I told my patients; the encouraging words I shared with fellow believers who were in distress; the motivational quotations I passed on to those who asked; and the prayers I lifted up to God on behalf of the sick and suffering I now reopened for personal scrutiny. It was now my turn to apply my beliefs to myself. Were those sentiments empty platitudes? Were the concepts practical? I rediscovered the benefits as I applied them conscientiously.

On one occasion my wife and I had been invited to meet with a Bible study group. We were asked to discuss James Dobson's book *When God Does Not Make Sense*. Part of our presentation included our own experience with chronic illness, since my wife had lived with Lupus for over twenty-two years at that time. I shared my reactions as her husband.

Now, I was the one with the illness. It was my turn to be the living witness. The lessons learned from studying the lives of Job, the Apostle Paul, and Naaman; the testimonies from friends and relatives who had suffered from various kinds of illness or loss; and my answered prayers. All served me well.

**"For this thing I besought the Lord thrice, that it might depart from me. And He said unto me, My grace is sufficient for thee: for My strength is made perfect in weakness. Most gladly therefore will I rather glory in my infirmities, that the power of Christ may rest upon me" (2 Corinthians 12:8, 9).**

## MIRROR

I took the time to review my life. I played the mental videotapes of events that were fresh in my mind as well as situations that were a little foggy from the remote past. In some areas I had matured, in others I had stagnated, and in others, yet, I had regressed.

This exercise reminded me of my psychiatry residency training. It was my professional duty to learn how to examine the lives and experiences of my patients in order to assist them with their emotional recovery and stability. Supervisory sessions were an integral part of my training. My skill of looking into the life history and related factors of the people under my care was like developing the art of using a psychological magnifying glass. However, all of the supervision did not focus on my skills. I also had personal sessions. The trainers examined me. I had to become aware of the circumstances that shaped my life and how those situations affected me as a person so that I would be able to better understand my patients. Those exercises were like looking into a mirror. I discovered that it was easier and considerably less threatening to focus on other people than to look at myself.

The analogy became relevant to my present condition. It was now my responsibility to learn from my experience and do what was necessary for me to recover as fully as possible.

**"Now therefore thus saith the LORD of hosts; Consider your ways" (Haggai 1:5).**

---

## MY FOURTH MIRACLE

I recently found myself reviewing several miraculous events in my life. I wondered how many times God intervened to spare my life. There were seven that I could enumerate. Accident-prone? Careless? Coincidence? Whatever the reason, God used the experiences to let me know that He had a protective hedge around me. I can recall seeing paintings of little children playing innocently close to danger and an angel on the scene protecting them from impending catastrophe. Perhaps that is what happened to me, repeatedly. One example, my fourth miracle, stands out above the others.

My family and I were traveling south on I-75 in Valdosta, Georgia. The road sign indicated that the right lane was closed ahead to allow for repaving, so I slowed down to accommodate the single lane of heavy traffic that was building up rapidly. In fact, it was building up too rapidly for me to avoid tailgating. The newly paved lane was now on my right glistening in the subtropical sun and announcing its presence further with the strong scent of fresh tar. I glanced at the rear view mirror just in time to see that an18-wheeler freight truck was bearing down behind us and getting uncomfortably larger and larger. My heart pounded furiously. It appeared to be located in my ears rather than in my chest. I sent up a quick prayer without words. I thought that the driver of the truck would do the opposite of whatever action I took. But, would he see my movement in time to know which way to turn in time to prevent running over us? Just then our car, the green and cream 1979 Riviera, turned left into the emergency lane and the 18-wheeler went the other way. I do not remember turning the steering wheel, for I froze in fear. However, I felt a pressure on my wrists. That was when our car escaped crashing into the vehicle ahead. An angel must have touched me. It took me half an hour to stop crying before we could continue our journey.

I cannot praise God enough for His undeserved favors. Now, He saved my life again.

**"The angel of the LORD encampeth round about them that fear him, and delivereth them" (Psalm 34:7).**

———◆◆◆———

## EXERCISE

During my youth, I attended a technical trade school for five years where regular physical exercise was a central part of the program. For four days a week we exercised on the campus, but on the fifth day we ran through the little town and frequently raced to the finish in order to get the best shower positions. Since that time I have exercised regularly and kept by body weight within a normal range. Now that I have retired and that my blood pressure is slightly elevated, it is imperative that I have a consistent exercise program. I used to observe people in the shopping mall who were there not to shop but to walk. How interesting! I would tell myself. Today I am part of that select group. Sometimes we greet each other; at other times we just walk oblivious to the other's concerns. I am happy that I had not said anything offensive or uncharitable about members of that universal club. Instead I would smile just to let them know that they were pleasantly noticed.

Now, I receive pleasant smiles and nods as I dodge the shoppers. I prefer, though, to exercise regularly at home as I have done throughout the years.

**"Therefore all things whatsoever ye would that men should do to you, do ye even so to them: for this is the law and the prophets" (Matthew 7:12).**

———◆◆◆———

## LISTEN

It became increasingly clear, during my reflective moments, that on many occasions I didn't listen attentively. As soon as I got the gist of what the other person was saying I formulated my response and delivered it. The context of the situation and the type of person to whom I was speaking determined what happened next. Sometimes, however, I recognized my error, apologized and made a midcourse correction. No doubt I have left countless bits of miscommunication in my relationships.

One benefit of my illness seemed to be that I was in a position to slow down some of the processes around me in order to learn from these mishaps. After all, what the other person has to say is just as important as my contribution. Not giving them my full attention was certainly inconsiderate, if not rude.

**"And be ye kind one to another, tenderhearted, forgiving one another, even as God for Christ's sake hath forgiven you" (Ephesians 4:32).**

---

## SANITARY CONCERNS

Initially I was embarrassed to shop in that section of stores where bladder control protection pads were on display. When I realized that I had to start purchasing these items I was hoping that they would be in an obscure section of the store. I had no such luck. When I finally located the pads I casually ventured to the spot. I would wait until the aisle was clear, look neither left nor right, make my selection and leave forthwith. In fact, on one occasion I asked my younger daughter, the educator, to purchase a package of the pads for me. She brought me a selection that appeared too feminine for me. I refused to use it. What did I expect?

Later, as I accepted my condition, I made my own purchases. I lingered in the aisles, compared brands, prices, and levels of absorbency. It no longer mattered to me who was aware of what I was doing in the store. Shopping for these items was to my benefit. Self-consciousness was secondary. I was finally comfortable with my condition.

**"For I am not ashamed of the gospel of Christ: for it is the power of God unto salvation to every one that believeth; to the Jew first, and also to the Greek" (Romans 1:16).**

## KELOID

My days for wearing revealing swim trunks that appeared to be sprayed on were long gone. Nevertheless I had not completely lost my vanity. I was concerned that when the midline (below the navel) suprapubic incision that was essential for my operation healed, a keloid would develop. Even if I wore the most modest swim trunk the scar would be exposed and a keloid would be more noticeable. The surgeon could give me no assurances, so I did not prolong this discussion with him. Besides, I wanted to keep my vanity to myself. At any rate, only time would tell what the outcome would be. I recalled that rubbing cocoa butter on the scar would reduce the likelihood of a keloid developing. As you may imagine I applied the salve faithfully.

Although the incision is completely healed a scar remains, but there is no keloid. It is a grim reminder of the ordeal I had to undergo or face death eventually from the cancer.

**"And one shall say unto him, What are these wounds in thine hands? Then he shall answer, Those with which I was wounded in the house of my friends "** **(Zechariah 13:6).**

## VULNERABILITY

The process of surgery placed me in an utterly vulnerable position. Despite the best efforts, the highest level of competency, or the state of alertness, something could go wrong. I was confident that members of my treatment team were trained to have a high index of suspicion if a threat to my stability arose. This thought reminded me of an experience my wife and I had when our second daughter was born.

We needed baby-sitting services and thought of a phone call we had received in response to the unsolicited newspaper announcement of our second daughter's birth in the small town where we lived. The call came from the Community Services Section of a recently relocated religious group. At that time I was on the Community Psychiatry rotation of my residency and met the leader of the group in my liaison contacts. His mission was to promote community improvement and comradery for all. His was an open door policy, and my wife and I attended one of his meetings. At a time of social unrest in the late 60's, that approach was a breath of fresh air. Finally, the whole community of believers would be united. That concept seemed reasonable and the approach an honest one. So with that in mind we called to accept the group's offer to baby-sit our little girls.

The representatives responded energetically, and passed our stringent screening interview. They did a good job. However, they emphatically refused to accept payment of any kind and even expressed their desire and willingness to serve us again. All we had to do was to call them. We thanked them for their generosity and parted company graciously. As they left, my wife and I knew that sooner or later we would have to pay in some form or another, perhaps beyond our control. We were uncomfortable with their generosity, and decided then and there not to call on them for further services. Ten years later, members of the group were involved in a mass suicide under their leader's command. We thanked God that He impressed us to avoid becoming involved with the group when we felt vulnerable.

**"For the LORD spake thus to me with a strong hand, and instructed me that I should not walk in the way of this people, ..." (Isaiah 8:11).**

---

## IMMUNITY

Seven months before I was aware that my benign prostate diagnosis had deteriorated into a malignant one I had a bout of chest pain. The initial screening examinations revealed no pathology; however, the concerned physician advised me to get a treadmill test in order to remove any doubts regarding possible heart disease. This was the second time I had this test, and it turned out to be within normal limits.

As the news of my condition spread, my wife received many calls. Many people were praying for my stability and were well aware of my lifestyle. One call stood out above the others. "What's Rudy doing having chest pains? We know he eats wisely. We look at what he eats. It is usually nutritious, and we make comments about it. He seemed to be in the best of health, too." The interesting implication about that call was that my lifestyle was supposed to protect me from illness, at least from heart disease. Although my heart was in good condition, the anticipated immunity did not transfer to another body system. I had to remind myself that all human beings, because of our sinful nature, would be subject to any ailment until sin and its tragic consequences are completely eradicated.

**"Beloved, I wish above all things that thou mayest prosper and be in health, even as thy soul prospereth" (3 John 1:2).**

## Nature: River Rocks I

The pace of my life slowed down considerably. Actually, I had little choice. I had heard it said that when you are flat on your back, it is hard not to look up. So I did not only look up, I looked around. I looked down. I discovered river rocks! They were everywhere! There were all kinds!
Smooth rocks.
　　Red rocks.
　　　　Yellow rocks.
　　　　　　Black rocks.
　　　　　　　White rocks.
　　　　　　　　Gray rocks.
　　　　　　　　　Oval rocks.
　　　　　　　　　　Flat rocks.
　　　　　　　　　　　Variegated rocks.
Following the urge to do something creative with these newly discovered objects, I washed and shellacked them. Surprisingly, my family accepted them as presents for decoration. Afterwards I discovered that river rocks were sold in stores. I had become too busy to observe some of the beauty and practical things that were all around. Not so with the shepherd boy, David. He knew where he could find smooth stones when he needed some.

**"And he took his staff in his hand, and chose him five smooth stones out of the brook, and put them in a shepherd's bag which he had, even in a scrip; and his sling was in his hand: and he drew near to the Philistine" (1 Samuel 17:40).**

## Leaks

It can be disastrous to ignore leaks, especially with the type of surgery I had. Because I had abdominal surgery, leakage was anticipated and planned for. Urine from my bladder that did not flow through the Foley catheter while my urethra was healing would escape into my abdominal cavity. If the urine is allowed to accumulate, a surgical emergency with tragic results was sure to take place. No surgeon wants that kind of complication, particularly when it can be avoided.

The solution was a Penrose drain as part of the basic operative plan. A stab incision was strategically made in my lower abdominal wall and a collapsible rubber tube inserted but anchored externally. This arrangement provided for the decreasing amount of urine that escaped into my abdominal cavity to drain out. When the drainage stopped the tube was no longer needed. My urologist cut the anchoring suture and removed the drain as planned. Thereafter the incision healed without complication.

The Plan of Redemption is just like that Penrose drain. The surgeon anticipated the possible problem and he provided the solution. Similarly, God knew that by creating Man with the power of choice, Man might sin. So at the foundation of the world the Back-up plan was established. God did not cancel His desire to make Man because he might sin. Instead, the Creator provided for the possibility. What a wise and loving God we serve!

**"And all that dwell upon the earth shall worship him, whose names are not written in the book of life of the Lamb slain from the foundation of the world" (Revelation 13:8).**

———◆———

## UNFINISHED BUSINESS

Many of my plans were curtailed as a result of my illness. The thought of unfinished business reminded me that, on one occasion, a jealous colleague referred to me as an "unfinished psychiatrist."

I had one more year of resident training in psychiatry to complete. The hospital administrator, however, appointed me as the director of a program instead of giving the responsibility to an available senior clinician. I had recently been trained in a new type of treatment for substance abusers, and on that basis the chief executive told me that my experience was invaluable. By establishing the program, drug abuse in the hospital environment would be minimized and patients would receive the specialized treatment they needed. I was new to that institution, but I had relevant experience. However, I had not completed my psychiatric training. My colleague was enraged about the choice and kept neither his opinions nor his feelings a secret. That was how I found out about his nickname for me. The hospital received statewide recognition for its contribution in this challenging field, and I relocated as previously planned to complete my training.

Now, at the close of my professional career, I'll have to shift my priorities and leave a number of issues for other psychiatrists to complete. The delivery of medical care is undergoing rapid changes. I'll just have to attend to the more critical issues of my health and not lament over unfinished healthcare reorganization.

**"Being confident of this very thing, that he which hath begun a good work in you will perform it until the day of Jesus Christ" (Philippians 1:6).**

———————◆◆◆———————

## LEGACY

Some time ago I saw an interesting Greeting Card for a Graduate. It contained a three-inch segment of a pencil and a note to the graduate stating that now was the time to "Make Your Mark on the World." I have read of people who gave instructions as to what they would like written on their tombstone. Then there are hosts of contributors who have made this world a better place to live in. Showers of accolades have been given to them–posthumously. When I reflect on the number of times I know my life has been spared (and the number of times I was not aware of how close I came to death), I thank God for His saving grace and wonder if I have accomplished the purpose for my life. I think of my legacy. What would my epitaph say? How would my eulogy read? What would people remember about me? Sobering thoughts these are. I hope that my legacy would be of a spiritual nature rather than a material one as was the case with the Israelite king, Hezekiah.

**"And he said, What have they seen in thine house? And Hezekiah answered, All the things that are in mine house have they seen: there is nothing among my treasures that I have not showed them. And Isaiah said unto Hezekiah, Hear the word of the LORD. Behold, the days come, that all that is in thine house, and that which thy fathers have laid up in store unto this day, shall be carried into Babylon: nothing shall be left, saith the LORD" (2 Kings 20:15-17).**

———————◆◆◆———————

## MEMORY

In the course of sharing experiences during my illness, I am finding out that there are some episodes for which I have no memory. I listen with interest about my behavior as various family members tell me what happened (at least to the best of their recollection). Some of the stories are humorous; some have to do with my need for medical care causing them to intervene for me. Under the influence of medication, I was able to carry out activities that were not permanently recorded in the memory pathways in my brain. It sounds like the behavior of an alcoholic during an episode of a "blackout." The action took place; others saw it; but the person has no memory of the event.

That is similar to what Jesus said He would do with our confessed sins. It would be as though we have never sinned.

**"And they shall teach no more every man his neighbour, and every man his brother, saying, Know the LORD: for they shall all know me, from the least of them unto the greatest of them, saith the LORD: for I will forgive their iniquity, and I will remember their sin no more" (Jeremiah 31:34).**

———◆——

## ANGER

I do not remember feeling angry. I clearly recall being edgy; hard to please; hard to get along with; and ill tempered. I could not bring myself to admit that what I just described were angry feelings. There was no particular focus or target: but looking back there is no doubt that what I just described was anger–plain and simple. I was complicating my life and that of the people around me. At times I retreated to my own private little world. After a while that method did not work. Sensing that I needed a change of scenery, I went to my "other world." I went to Trinidad. I shifted the focus from myself to family members whom I had not seen for several years, and saw how a group of visually impaired people conducted a fund-raising program, among other activities. That journey helped tremendously, but I still had to come to grips with my feelings.

**"Be ye angry, and sin not: let not the sun go down upon your wrath" (Ephesians 4:26).**

## LAUGHTER

It was difficult for me to have a really good laugh during the first few days after my operation. Instinctively I would hold back the laughter and support my lower abdomen with my hands. Fortunately, my wife had given me a stuffed teddy bear, Miss Huggabie, when I had an earlier operation. It came in handy again. Visitors usually were amused and surprised to see my toy; it seemed so out of character for me, but it worked. I could laugh heartier if I could control the abdominal pressure by holding the cuddly toy against my abdomen until my incision healed.

**"A merry heart doeth good like a medicine: but a broken spirit drieth the bones" (Proverbs 17:22).**

## AIRPLANES

The long months of my convalescence accentuated my need to be with members of my family in Trinidad whom I had not seen for almost four years. I wanted to reassure them that I was recovering satisfactorily. The real truth was that when I spoke to some of them they did not know who I was. That was heartbreaking. So I had to visit them, and at the same time, I could test how I was recuperating.

I arrived and settled down to a modest routine of visits and periods of rest. Then on that fateful Tuesday morning of September 11, 2001, one week after my arrival in Trinidad, television pictures of airplanes deliberately crashing into the New York World Trade Center, the Pentagon, and an open field in Pennsylvania stunned the free world. Pictures of billowing clouds of horror overshadowed the idyllic tropical skies of sunny Trinidad. I watched in dismay. Discontent from the East attacked the symbols of affluence and democracy from the West. Airplanes, instruments of progress and advance of knowledge, became tools of vengeance and terror. The scenes were not those of cinematography at its best: they were real. What a wake-up call that was! While I was on my private mission of family unity and recovery from my illness, there were other people who made horrific international demonstrations of their obsession with divisiveness and intolerance.

**"Beat your plowshares into swords, and your pruninghooks into spears: let the weak say, I am strong. Assemble yourselves, and come, all ye heathen, and**

**gather yourselves together round about: thither cause thy mighty ones to come down, O LORD" (Joel 3:10, 11).**

---

## BABY-SIT

Prior to my surgery, our older daughter and her husband decided to relocate near to us. She did not want their children to be deprived of having grandparents nearby as it was with her. When the time came, she asked us to be available to baby-sit and we agreed enthusiastically. Meanwhile, I had my episode with surgery. When I arrived home from the hospital my family gathered around my bed and placed my grandson next to me. I suddenly realized that the six-month old bundle of joy was not going to be a passive receptacle of our love and concern. He loved us, too; but he expressed it with energetic bounces, little regard for where he pushed his unco-ordinated hands and feet, wanting to be held, perpetual motion, and unannounced needs for frequent diaper changes, among others. I was simply not prepared to give the constant attention he needed, and, at that time, neither was my wife.

Just then, we discovered that a cousin was coming to visit. Her usual trips were in the summer. However, her plans changed: she would be taking her "holidays" differently on this occasion. Best of all she was available when we needed someone to baby-sit our grandson. How convenient! Just when we needed someone to care for our grandson in our place, God provided a family member.

**"Then Abraham lifted his eyes and looked, and there behind him was a ram caught in a thicket by its horns. So Abraham went and took the ram, and offered it up for a burnt offering instead of his son. And Abraham called the name of the place, The-Lord-Will-Provide; as it is said to this day, 'In the Mount of the Lord it shall be provided'" (Genesis 22: 13, 14, NKJV).**

## JOY

Not every day was a bad day. I was happy to be alive. I felt joyful about the improvement in my condition. I could do things that healthy people took for granted. I can remember the first time I dangled my feet on the right side of the hospital bed, unhooked the Foley catheter bag which hung from the bed frame, steadied the portable I.V. pole, stepped off the bed, secured the bow at the back of my gown, ambled out of my room, and walked pass the Nurses' Station unassisted. That sequence was a small step but, nevertheless, a great accomplishment. I was on my way to recovery! That was joy!

**"For His anger is but for a moment, His favor is for life; Weeping may endure for a night, but joy comes in the morning" (Psalms 30:5, NKJV).**

## TURNING POINT

A number of incidents took place in quick succession and brought my reaction to my condition into focus for me. One day, while I was assisting my wife in the grocery store I became tearful. I left the store immediately. On another occasion we had a problem with ants in one of the kitchen cupboards. Our younger daughter, the educator, assessed the situation and came up with a solution before I could even figure out what was going on. I quietly excused myself and walked away feeling useless. Next, a dear friend and colleague called on the phone from out-of-town. My family told me who was calling, and I simply ignored the information and refused to talk to him. Later, I went to keep a dental appointment, and I cried in the dentist's chair when she asked how I was doing.

I remember thinking, "So this is what it is like to be a patient. The illness is controlling me, and I am just going along with it." This series of events jolted me. I did not like where I was headed, and I needed to turn around quickly.

**"And Peter answered him and said, 'Lord, if it be thou, bid me come unto thee on the water'. And he said, 'Come'. And when Peter was come down out of the ship, he walked on the water, to go to Jesus. But when he saw the wind boisterous, he was afraid; and beginning to sink, he cried, saying, 'Lord, save me' " (Matthew 14:28-30).**

# HOME

I felt homesick. It was time to go home. Nothing could prevent me from going. That's what I did. Off to Trinidad I went. On the plane I saw all the people I wanted to see; went all the places I wanted to go; ate all the delicious mangoes and succulent sapodillas I wanted to eat; and sang all the favorite hymns I wanted to sing. I relished the balmy breezes and swaying coconut palm trees only to realize that I was daydreaming.

I opened my eyes just in time to disembark. I was home. In the customs line I could not ignore the sudden jolts of reality. Reality? To which home would my driver take me? I had to ponder several options. One possibility was New Jersey, La Brea, my address when I was single and left the island 44 years earlier; or Railroad Avenue, the address when I returned with my wife and one child and another on the way ten years later. I had other choices, including the various locations of my childhood years, now occupied by several members of my family.

Friends had relocated: some went to England, Canada, the USA, and some to other parts of the thriving island. A few friends remained local. They had aged almost beyond recognition, but they would know me. After all, I had not changed except for my Americanized accent. So I thought.

I would have to decide with which family members would I eat boiled plantain, taste yellow yam, sip a sweet drink (soda), and spend a night. Then there would be choices about locations for church attendance and visits to former places of work and schools attended (energy permitting).

Sooner or later my trip would end. I would have to cease trading youthful stories and prepare to return – home.

This journey, filled with entwined memories and fantasies, made me realize the lack of permanence in my earthly abode. The spiritual reality stimulated deeper concerns of my past, present, and future. It turned my thoughts toward heaven where home will have a meaning that the human mind cannot now conceive.

**"But as it is written, Eye hath not seen, nor ear heard, neither have entered into the heart of man, the things which God hath prepared for them that love him" (1 Corinthians 2:9).**

## TREASURES

I was browsing through some books in my home library when it occurred to me that when I die some kind of disposition would have to be made of my informative volumes. In fact the same thing would have to be done with my precious memorabilia and whatever I owned. Think of it, my treasures might be another person's junk. I could remember where I purchased certain books and the reasons for adding them to my collection. I reviewed mental travelogues of my trips to various parts of the world. I especially like the slide of a nameless person looking out of a window in Buckingham Palace. Two other favorite slides are scenes of Robben Island as seen from Table Mountain in Cape Town, South Africa, and the tunnels of Cu Chi in Viet Nam. Further, documents I saved since my youth give pictorial accounts of my life, with each item telling its own fascinating story.

All of these items played a part in what I had become. But they are materialistic. They are temporal. As I continued to recuperate, I wondered if I would maintain the deep spiritual experience I was enjoying or if I would return to business as usual when the distress was over.

**"Lay not up for yourselves treasures upon earth, where moth and rust doth corrupt, and where thieves break through and steal: But lay up for yourselves treasures in heaven, where neither moth nor rust doth corrupt, and where thieves do not break through nor steal: For where your treasure is, there will your heart be also" (Matthew 6:19-21).**

## TEARS

My tears flowed easily at times whether the triggers were internal or external. Mainly, I was happy to be alive. So I cried because of joy. When it dawned on me that I survived the operation and that the cancer was no longer in my body, I cried. When I found out that the blood test at my first office follow-up visit showed no trace of malignant prostate activity, I cried.

At a family reunion picnic, nine months into my recuperation, a cousin commented that it was difficult to imagine that I looked in such good shape for someone who had been through so much. I cried. He meant it as a compliment, but I suddenly burst into tears. Another cousin nearby encouraged me to let the tears flow. She watched me closely then waited patiently until I stopped crying and said, "Now, don't you feel better?" I looked at my wife who sat nearby. Finally, I nodded my head in silent acknowledgement of the heartfelt support. Until then I had participated bravely in various activities for several days. I had given myself private compliments for being in control during the festivities. We were now at a public beach in Miami on the Sunday afternoon reminiscing, playing games, eating, and swimming. What a time to cry!

As I have recovered over the past two years I have had fewer and fewer episodes of spontaneous crying both publicly and privately.

**"And God shall wipe away all tears from their eyes; and there shall be no more death, neither sorrow, nor crying, neither shall there be any more pain: for the former things are passed away" (Revelation 21:4).**

## MENTORING

Countless persons helped to shape my life: many of them unknowingly. Now, as I reflected in silent gratitude, I wondered how many lives I had helped to shape. Once, I attempted to join a Boys and Girls Club. Somehow, I did not seem to fit in, so I dropped out. My interest in becoming a mentor, however, did not wane. I prayed silently to the Lord for direction. Then one day it happened. The person came to me, but it took many years for me to recognize what was happening. How strange!

I was busy photographing scenes at a youth rally in Trinidad. The sun was hot and there was little shade. Somehow I had the eerie feeling that someone was close by. I looked around, aimed the camera, and clicked spontaneously. An enterprising little girl had found a cool spot–in my shadow. A shadow in the scene was obvious when I developed the photograph, but that technical detail did not matter. I could not forget her face, though. When I saw her eight years later on another visit and asked her about the incident she had no idea what I was talking about, but her mother remembered. Smart mother! She kept up with the whereabouts of her daughter and did not forget the encounter. I sent them an enlargement of the photograph, and I still did not recognize the potential of our fleeting contacts. To my pleasant surprise her "thank you" response included a request for me to be her mentor. That is how God works. He allows our paths to cross and our lives to intersect according to His timetable. It is our task to recognize these incidents for what they are worth.

**"Train up a child in the way he should go: and when he is old, he will not depart from it" (Proverbs 22:6).**

## HELL

In May 2001 I went to Hell. It was hot but I enjoyed it. And when I met two persons who turned out to be members of my worldwide Church, I was even happier. At first we were strangers, but as we got to know each other, we hugged, we smiled, and we traded experiences. I was so happy I did not want to leave. Okay, what's the gag? I am referring, of course, to a brief encounter in Hell, Grand Cayman Island, which was one of the stops on a vacation cruise. I met the proprietors of a gift shop, and we were having so much fun getting acquainted that I almost missed the tourist transportation for the rest of the tour and back to the ship.

When I mentioned Hell at first, I am sure you became concerned because of its negative connotation. Then I gave more information, which caused you to change your initial thoughts and reaction. Most likely, you initially projected your biases onto my words and thereafter had to make the necessary adjustments as I clarified myself. I can imagine that is what happened to the Samaritan woman who met Jesus at the well when they talked about water. She used the same word as He did but they applied different meanings. However, Jesus knew what her basic need was.

**"The woman said to Him, 'Sir, You have nothing to draw with, and the well is deep. Where then do You get that living water?' " (John 4:11, NKJV)**

## ACCIDENTS

There are five accidents that I can remember in which I could have died, were it not for God's providence. Two involved automobiles, two involved falls and one involved an averted drowning. At times I wonder if I am accident-prone. Then came the episode with the malignancy.

Six weeks after my operation, Elisa, one of my goddaughters, was killed in a car accident. We were devastated. Here was a young lady with a full life ahead of her. I had talked to her two weeks earlier and her ambition was to make a difference wherever she went. She had just left one community activity and was heading to her university campus for a Bible study session when her life ended.

How does God decide which life to spare and which one to allow to be taken away? Is that even the question to ask? This situation is one that the human mind cannot fully comprehend. Whatever answer we give raises a few others that are more puzzling than the original one.

**"Then they that feared the LORD spake often one to another: and the LORD hearkened, and heard it, and a book of remembrance was written before him for them that feared the LORD, and that thought upon his name" (Malachi 3:16).**

---

## LIFE'S LENSES

I often thought about the reasons that make people with the same illness look at it quite differently. For that matter, it might be a situation in which one person feels hopeful and the other person feels hopeless. This puzzling situation happened to me on a number of occasions.

The other person and I looked at the same situation and came to completely different conclusions. Why does this phenomenon exist? The field of optometry/ophthalmology can help to explain. Here the manner in which lenses affect vision is one such example. Concave lenses make objects appear shorter. Convex lenses make objects appear larger. The shape of the eye is also important, as is the distance between the eye and the object being viewed.

The emotional experiences we have had determine the way we see and understand the world. They shape our emotional lenses. Our past encounters remain with us and give meaning to our present and projections to our future. I have heard it said that the past is always present, and that the past is prologue. If I were to carry the analogy of the lenses further, I would suggest that there are social, psychological, and spiritual counterparts to myopia, hyperopia, presbyopia, astigmatism, cataracts, and blindness.

**"Lo, mine eye hath seen all this, mine ear hath heard and understood it. What ye know, the same do I know also: I am not inferior unto you. Your remembrances are like unto ashes, your bodies to bodies of clay" (Job 13:1, 2, 12).**

# COLOR INSERTS:
# SELF-DIRECTED OCCUPATIONAL
# THERAPY ITEMS

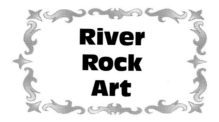

**River
Rock
Art**

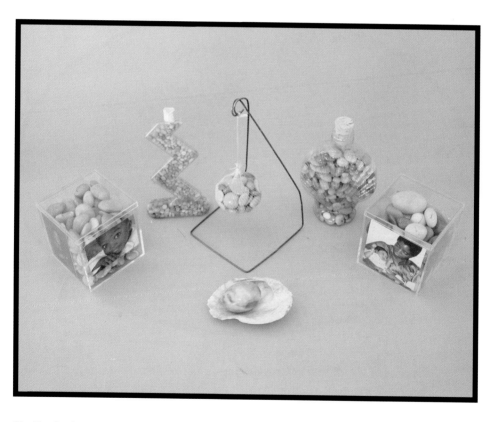

*Shellacked river rocks used for paperweights, photo displays, or other decorations.*

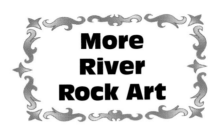

# More River Rock Art

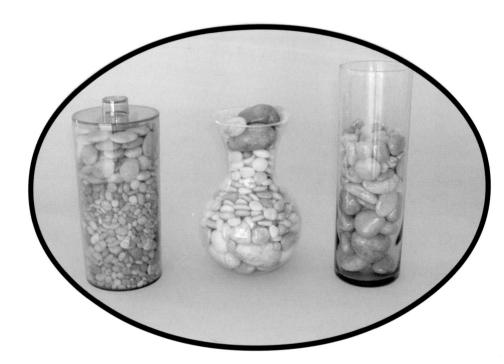

*Assorted shellacked river rocks in plastic or glass containers.*
*The rock collecting experience also inspired devotional selections.*

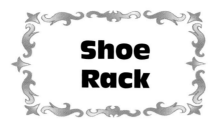

# Shoe
# Rack

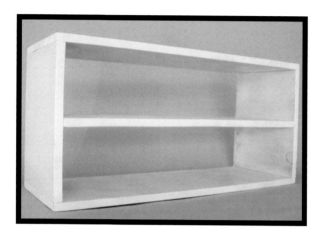

*My woodworking experience became useful. Shoeracks prevent shoe clutter at front and rear doorways.*

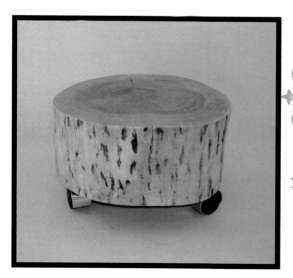

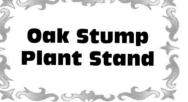

# Oak Stump
# Plant Stand

*This discarded oak stump from a construction site was converted into a plant stand on wheels.*

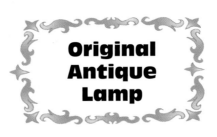

# Original Antique Lamp

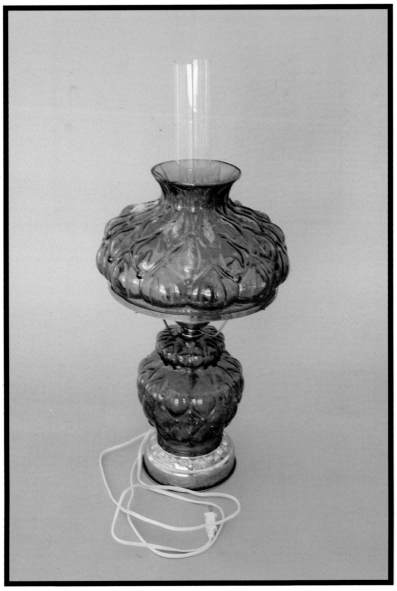

*(Before) Antique lamp with nonfunctioning electrical parts.*

43

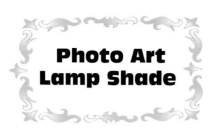

# Photo Art
# Lamp Shade

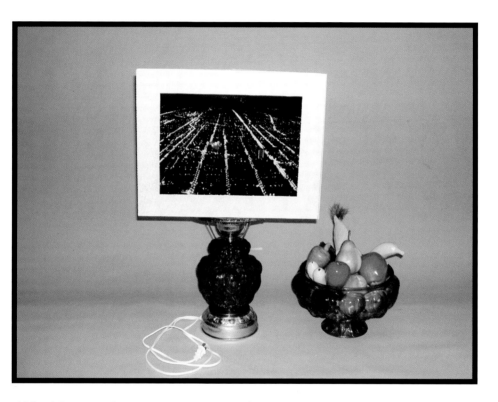

*(After) Lamp with contemporary triangular photo frame shade [city of Chicago]
and fruit bowl made from the original lampshade.*

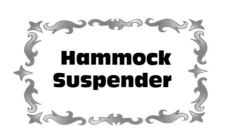

# Hammock Suspender

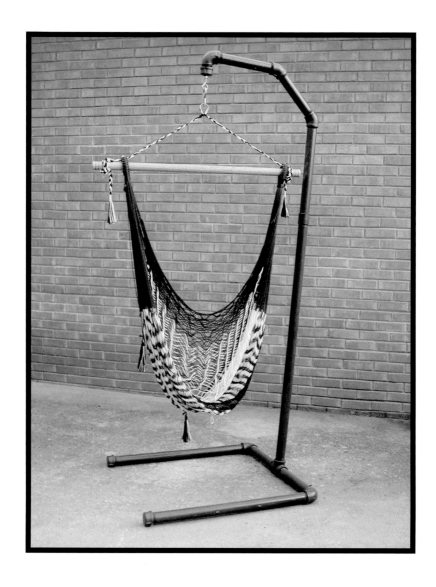

*Moveable hammock frame was constructed from metal pipes. It allows for relocation when desired.*

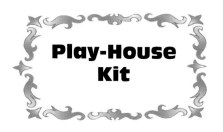

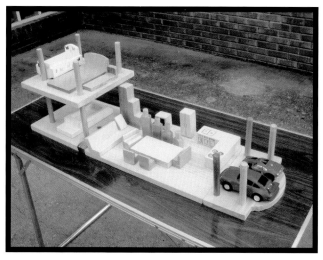

*Easy assembly. Made from scraps of wood. [except cars]*

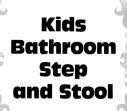

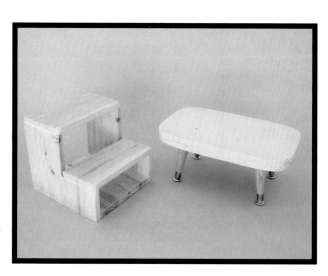

*Simple wood items for convenient use—to add height when needed.*

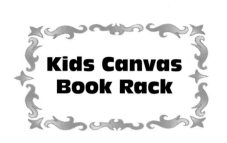

# Kids Canvas Book Rack

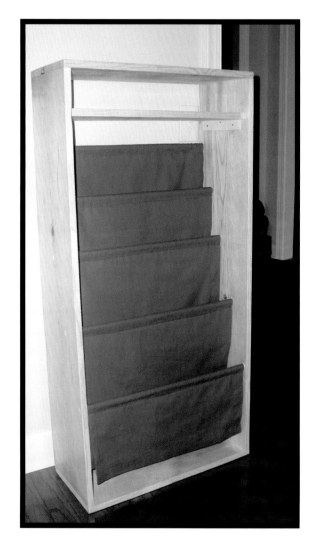

*Canvas pockets afford easier access to books and less attention required for neatness compared to stacked shelves. Top and upper shelf provide for storage of other items.*

# PART I (continued)

———◆———

## CHANGE

I stood breathless for what seemed like an eternity. The scenery had changed. Something was missing. It was no longer there! Did it have to go? Change was the price of progress. I could have tried to save it and risk being laughed at. I knew the answers to all the rhetorical questions I could pose. I would have raised futile objections. The new building needed the space and the magnolia tree was in the way. Once the decision had been made to modernize the facility, the avalanche of renovation decisions could not stop. In just a few minutes the obedient bulldozer leveled scores of years of growth and silent beauty. Now the tree was gone!

The stately magnolia tree whose picturesque flowers chronicled the seasons was my favorite landmark outside of my office. I had a ritual: unlock the office; lay my attaché case on the desk; don my lab coat; open the window shutters; admire the magnolia tree and look for the seasonal changes of the magnificent flowers; turn away; sit at my desk; get to work. The routine varied only when the phone rang or some urgent item interrupted me.

I did not cry! At least no tears flowed. I really missed that tree. When I recovered, I reflected on the numerous changes that were taking place in the delivery of health care. Some contestants in the management/provider conflict referred to the new approach as "managed money" instead of "managed care." I wasn't handling the changes adequately and, although I knew better intellectually, over a period of several years, I allowed the stress to escalate into distress.

**"To every thing there is a season, and a time to every purpose under the heaven: A time to be born, and a time to die; a time to plant, and a time to pluck up that which is planted; A time to kill, and a time to heal; a time to break down, and a time to build up; A time to weep, and a time to laugh; a time to mourn, and a time to dance" (Ecclesiastes 3:1-4).**

## NATURE: RIVER ROCKS II

I was recovering quite well and went out one day to collect river rocks.
Suddenly I identified with the ones I did not select.

From riverbed to riverbank
Washed from place to place without a choice
Absorbing the color of the environment,
My rough edges smoothed out by the unwilling turbulence.

Overpowered by the constant flow,
Picked up and thrown back,
Picked up and polished,
Picked up and stored but never used as planned,
I awaited other choices.

Crouched as gravel for sidewalks and parking lots,
Crushed, bruised and displaced by progress,
I wonder what next!

Ah! Decoration for water art!
Unique, special, incognito,
Flat, round, oval,
Small, medium, large,
Black, white, pink, gray, red, yellow, variegated, and speckled,
I reveled quietly in the possibilities.

Oh, No! Don't paint me over,
If you could only hear me!
Let me take my place
On hills or vales, wastelands or oases and await
Appreciation.

**"And God saw every thing that he had made, and, behold, it was very good. And the evening and the morning were the sixth day" (Genesis 1:31).**

## NATURE: RIVER ROCKS III

In addition to writing about my experiences, I engaged in a number of activities for my self-styled "occupational therapy." Interestingly, I gave words to inanimate objects through which I also expressed my inner concerns. The Biblical account of David's five smooth stones gave me this outlet.

Stone 1.　"The shepherd boy stepped into the clear stream and picked me up the moment he laid eyes on me. Look at my shape. I am perfect for a sling. I'll never miss the mark."

Stone 2.　"You may have the appearance of success, but you'll need more than that. I came from a family of achievers. I have pedigree. I'm the one."

Stone 3.　"I don't have the features I've heard mentioned so far. You cannot see my advantages. My importance is my potential. My value is hidden until I am released. Now, think about that."

Stone 4.　"You guys should hear yourselves. You sound typically macho. I may be small in size, but it will take a woman with my accomplishments to bring down the giant. No man can resist me. That's why I'm here."

Stone 5.　"I am just honored to be one of the five. Wherever I am I try to do my best. There is nothing about me that is particularly outstanding except a Power that comes over me when there is a job to be done. If I am put into the sling when the time comes, I want to be guided to hit the mark."

**"And he took his staff in his hand, and chose him five smooth stones out of the brook, and put them in a shepherd's bag which he had, even in a scrip; and his sling was in his hand: and he drew near to the Philistine" (1 Samuel 17:40).**

# THE SOUND MIND

Throughout my career as a psychiatrist, I compared psychological principles with what the Holy Bible had to say about life. I thought that since God made us He had to have an operating manual somewhere. So that's how I viewed the Scriptures. That being the case, it should not be surprising to find laws and guidelines for human behavior there. One of the cardinal aspects of mental functioning is the psychoanalytic concept of id, ego, and super ego. Because this view was accompanied by theories that seemed far-fetched, it was found objectionable to many people within as well as outside psychological circles.

Laws of mental functioning were described long before modern principles of the mind were articulated. Consider the id as basic power. Think of the ego as capacity to choose. Look at the super ego as the conscience. Fear, including anxiety, worry, and depression, then, is the state of disharmony between the parts of our thinking faculties. This concept is surely not a new one.

In applying this principle to myself I wondered what went wrong. I wanted to make sure that, in the future, my health had some sense of balance. Whether I use terms such as id, ego, and superego or whether I speak of body, mind, and spirit, God's desire for me is balance. Looking back, I had been preoccupied with morbid distractions and suffered the consequences. The task for me now is to apply consistently the laws of nature and spirituality and position myself to reap the preventive benefits. I can say without a doubt that this approach has hastened and stabilized my recovery.

**"For God has not given us a spirit of fear, but of power and of love and of a sound mind" (2 Timothy 1:7, NKJV).**

## DISTRACTIONS

On a hot summer day in 1961 I combed the streets of Hinsdale, Illinois, in pursuit of customers who would purchase the magazines I sold for a religious publishing company. I met a young couple that listened intently. The expression on their faces puzzled me for a while, and I was almost distracted from my presentation. I wondered if the reason was their fascination with my foreign accent. So I adjusted my speech by telling them that their purchase of a single copy or a subscription of one or several of the magazines would benefit them and at the same time help to finance of my medical school education. I kept on speaking, and they kept on looking at each other. Finally the young lady broke their silence. Gazing longingly at her companion she said, "Honey, we should return to dental school and finish. We've been away too long." They stated that they had been on the campus where I was headed and had dropped out for reasons that they did not share. Our brief contact on that torrid day jolted them back on track.

Like that lovely couple, I may have had good reasons for being distracted. Intellectually, I knew all of the benefits of a balanced life. But somewhere along the way, I lost focus. The cancer experience woke me up. At any rate, it is my prayer that the way I have dealt with it is a living witness of God's extravagant grace.

**"But take heed to yourselves, lest your hearts be weighed down with carousing, drunkenness, and cares of this life, and that Day come on you unexpectedly." (Luke 21:34, NKJV).**

## TOGETHERNESS

Trust in God, support from family and friends, paying close attention to basic laws of health, maintaining a positive outlook, acknowledging setbacks and knowing how to deal with them, and sharing my experience have gone a long way to help me to accept my human frailties. I am living a satisfied life without a prostate gland – to which Ambroise Paré referred as the "gate keeper"– but with neurological functions preserved. My wife has survived for over twenty-seven years with the ups and downs of Systemic Lupus Erythematosus, and, as a spouse at close range, I have learned from how she copes. Our basic schedule is one of being active when her illness is in relative remission and slowing down to rest when there is a flare up.

Now we balance our activities in tandem with each other for mutual support. Indeed we are discovering the true meaning of being a help meet to each other. Each day calls for new adjustment to frustration and disappointments with tolerance, acceptance, and patience. I write further about these experiences in Part II, Poetry and Prose. As I expected, the Holy Bible, God's handbook for mankind, had already given insight on this topic of togetherness. It described how the human body and organizations accommodate for loss of parts by cooperating for the success of the unit.

**"But now are they many members, yet but one body. And the eye cannot say unto the hand, I have no need of thee: nor again the head to the feet, I have no need of you. And whether one member suffer, all the members suffer with it; or one member be honoured, all the members rejoice with it. Now ye are the body of Christ, and members in particular" (1 Corinthians 12: 20, 21, 26, 27).**

## REJOICE

Ordinarily, I express myself in a modest manner–whether the occasion calls for exuberance or lamentation. However, the experiences of these past two years have exposed me to a wider variety of emotions in their fullest form. I reflect on my stormy silence the moment I heard my diagnosis for the first time. Although I was aware of that possibility, the protective purpose of denial postponed the depth of my hurt until I received confirmation from the pathologist.

Later, the thought of death made me search my soul with unfamiliar passion. But because I have a continued relationship with God, my fears did not deteriorate into despair. When I awoke from the anesthesia and saw my family at my bedside I rejoiced, although my quiet joy was further subdued by my medicated condition. (I can understand how easy it is for a person to become addicted to narcotics.)

From time to time, with decreasing frequency, I cried without warning, both from depression and the joy of being alive, and as the two-year mark of my survival approached, I rejoiced. I was alive! I was recovering! Best of all I was writing about it! Perhaps that was what the Apostle Paul meant by "glorying in infirmities."

**"But we have this treasure in earthen vessels, that the excellency of the power may be of God, and not of us. We are troubled on every side, yet not distressed; we are perplexed, but not in despair; Persecuted, but not forsaken; cast down, but not destroyed" (2 Corinthians 4:7-9).**

# PART II: POETRY AND PROSE

## PRAYERS

## Prayer for Guidance

*One of my favorite ministers once stated that we should be careful what we pray for. He added that often God grants our requests, and then we tell Him that's not what we meant. This seven-part Prayer for Guidance is intended to provide a balanced focus that includes our relationship with our fellow man and our readiness to meet Our Heavenly Father.*

Father, help me to know Your will for my life.

Please bring to my attention whatever I need in order to successfully meet the challenges of this life and to get ready for Jesus' coming. You've answered my prayers in the past, and I know that You'll answer me now.

Please don't let what You reveal scare me. I know that I've downplayed some things I've done and even forgotten others. There are also things that I should have done that I didn't do.

If I can't handle by myself what you show me, please send some assistance and help me to recognize it. I want to keep the channels open.

Please help me to get it right early and not have to go through the turmoil to change too many times. I know that depends on me, so help me yield to You.

Help me to remember that others are struggling too. Help me not to become haughty. Help me not to become self-righteous as though I've never sinned. Make me sensitive to others.

Finally, Father, thank You for Your concern. When You take the time to answer my prayers, the least I could do is to be grateful.

In the precious name of Jesus, AMEN....

# Sufficient Grace

One month after I underwent a radical prostatectomy for adenocarcinoma, I realized I had not seriously questioned God about my plight. I was experiencing urinary incontinence, one of the complications of the surgical procedure, and I responded to the urge to go to the bathroom in the wee hours one morning. I thought that was the perfect time to have a little talk with Jesus.

It was my intent to raise some questions. The past four weeks had sped by too rapidly. Had I been in denial? I had not even fully formulated any questions in my mind as I got out of bed. When I reached the bathroom, I found myself saying, *"My Grace is sufficient for you" (2 Cor. 12:9, NKJV)*. My desire to formulate questions disappeared immediately. I relaxed in response to those comforting words. So much for my little talk with Jesus! The answer came before I could ask the question.

Two weeks later, my goddaughter, Elisa, was killed in an automobile accident. I was devastated. Although it was risky for me to travel, my wife and I decided to attend the funeral. Our grief would have been worse if we did not go. At that time I tired easily and I could not manage our luggage very well. To make matters worse, the young lady who came to pick us up at the airport gladly and effortlessly took care of the suitcases. I pondered my condition in the back seat of the car, and I wept bitterly. Pretty macho, huh!

My wife reached back to me from the front seat and whispered, " We are almost there. Remember you have to be strong. We have to see how Jeremy (the teen-age brother of the deceased) is holding out."

I desperately and silently appealed to the Lord for guidance. Again, the words came, "My grace is sufficient for you." But I was not satisfied. I wanted something more personal. Then the Holy Spirit whispered, **"Try 'God's grace is sufficient for me.' "** I did and calmed down immediately. Since that time, I usually personalize the statement with the mnemonic, **G.G.I.S.F.M.**

# HOLY SCRIPTURES

## Communion

*This responsive reading (for the congregation or a speech choir) is a collection of Old Testament prophecies and their fulfillment in the New Testament.*

Behold my servant, whom I uphold; mine elect, in whom my soul delighteth; I have put my spirit upon him: he shall bring forth judgment to the Gentiles. (Isa. 42:1)

**He riseth from supper, and laid aside his garments; and took a towel, and girded himself. (John 13:4)**

And one shall say unto him, What are these wounds in thine hands? Then he shall answer, Those with which I was wounded in the house of my friends. (Zech. 13:6)

**Then Judas, which betrayed him, answered and said, Master, is it I? He said unto him, Thou hast said. (Matt. 26:25)**

And thus ye shall eat it; with your loins girded, your shoes on your feet, and your staff in your hand; and ye shall eat it in haste: it is the Lord's Passover. (Ex. 12:11)

**And as they were eating, Jesus took bread, and blessed it, and break it, and gave it to the disciples, and said, Take, eat; this is my body. (Matt. 26:26)**

He was oppressed, and he was afflicted, yet he openeth not his mouth: he is brought as a lamb to the slaughter, and as a sheep before her shearers is dumb, so he openeth not his mouth. (Isa. 53:7)

**And he took the cup, and gave thanks, and gave it to them, saying, Drink ye all of it. (Matt. 26:27)**

And I will put enmity between thee and the woman, and between thy seed and her seed; it shall bruise thy head, and thou shalt bruise his heel. (Gen. 3:15)

**For this is my blood of the new testament, which is shed for many for the remission of sins. (Matt. 26:28)**

He shall call to the heavens from above, and to the earth, that he may judge his people. Gather my saints together unto me; those that have made a covenant with me by sacrifice. (Psalm 50:4, 5)

**But I say unto you, I will not drink henceforth of this fruit of the vine, until that day when I drink it new with you in my Father's kingdom. (Matt. 26: 29)**

Let the wilderness and the cities thereof lift up their voice (Isa. 42:11). He shall see of the travail of his soul, and shall be satisfied (Isa. 53:11). He will make an utter end: affliction shall not rise up the second time. (Nahum 1:9)

**And when they had sung an hymn, they went out into the Mount of Olives. (Matt. 26:30)**

———————◆◆◆◆———————

# The Twenty-Third Psalm

A Responsive Reading for a Speech Choir

**Leader**: THE LORD IS MY SHEPHERD;

**Choir:**  I am the good shepherd, and know my sheep, and am known of mine. As the Father knoweth me, even so know I the Father: and I lay down my life for the sheep. (John 10:14, 15)

**Leader**: I SHALL NOT WANT.

**Choir:**  But my God shall supply all your need according to His riches in glory by Christ Jesus. (Philippians 4:19)

**Leader**: HE MAKETH ME TO LIE DOWN IN GREEN PASTURES:

**Choir:**   When thou liest down, thou shalt not be afraid: yea, thou shalt lie down, and thy sleep shall be sweet. (Proverbs 3:24)

**Leader**: HE LEADETH ME BESIDE THE STILL WATERS.

**Choir:**   Thus saith the Lord, thy Redeemer, the Holy One of Israel; I am the Lord thy God which teacheth thee to profit, which leadeth thee by the way that thou shouldest go.  (Isaiah 48:17)

**Leader**: HE RESTORETH MY SOUL:

**Choir:**   Restore unto me the joy of thy salvation; and uphold me with thy free spirit. (Psalm 51:12)

**Leader**: HE LEADETH ME IN THE PATHS OF RIGHTEOUSNESS FOR HIS NAME'S SAKE.

**Choir:**   And thine ears shall hear a word behind thee, saying, This is the way, walk ye in it, when ye turn to the right hand, and when ye turn to the left. (Isaiah 30:21)

**Leader**: YEA, THOUGH I WALK THROUGH THE VALLEY OF THE SHADOW OF DEATH, I WILL FEAR NO EVIL:

**Choir:**   Fear thou not; for I am with thee: be not dismayed; for I am thy God: I will strengthen thee; yea, I will help thee; yea, I will uphold thee with the right hand of my righteousness.  (Isaiah 41:10)

**Leader**: FOR THOU ART WITH ME;

**Choir:**  For he hath said, I will never leave thee, nor forsake thee. (Hebrews 13:5)

**Leader**: THY ROD AND THY STAFF THEY COMFORT ME.

**Choir:**  We are troubled on every side, yet not distressed; we are perplexed, but not in despair; Persecuted, but not forsaken; cast down, but not destroyed. (2 Corinthians 4:8, 9)

**Leader**: THOU PREPAREST A TABLE BEFORE ME IN THE PRESENCE OF MINE ENEMIES:

**Choir:**  For He shall give His angels charge over thee, to keep thee is all thy ways. They shall bear thee up in their hands, lest thou dash thy foot against a stone.  (Psalms 91:11, 12)

**Leader**: THOU ANOINTEST MY HEAD WITH OIL;

**Choir:**  But ye are a chosen generation, a royal priesthood, an holy nation, a peculiar people; that ye should shew forth the praises of Him who hath called you out of darkness into his marvelous light. (1 Peter 2:9)

**Leader**: MY CUP RUNNETH OVER.

**Choir:**  And I will make them and the places round about my hill a blessing; and I will cause the shower to come down in his season; there shall be showers of blessing. (Ezekiel 34:26)

**Leader**: SURELY GOODNESS AND MERCY SHALL FOLLOW ME ALL THE DAYS OF MY LIFE:

**Choir:**  I have been young, and now am old; yet have I not seen the righteous forsaken, nor his seed begging bread. (Psalms 37:25)

**Leader**: AND I WILL DWELL IN THE HOUSE OF THE LORD FOREVER.

**Choir:**  Then we which are alive and remain shall be caught up together with them in the clouds, to meet the Lord in the air: and so shall we ever be with the Lord. (1 Thess. 4:17)

# The Lord's Prayer

A Responsive Reading
Based on
(Matthew 6: 9-13)

**Our Father which art in heaven,**

"Wherefore David blessed the LORD before all the congregation: and David said, Blessed be thou, LORD God of Israel our father, for ever and ever. Thine, O LORD, is the greatness, and the power, and the glory, and the victory, and the majesty: for all that is in the heaven and in the earth is thine; thine is the kingdom, O LORD, and thou art exalted as head above all. Both riches and honour come of thee, and thou reignest over all; and in thine hand is power and might; and in thine hand it is to make great, and to give strength unto all "
(1 Chronicles 29: 10-12).

**Hallowed be Thy name.**

"Then the Levites, Jeshua, and Kadmiel, Bani, Hashabniah, Sherebiah, Hodijah, Shebaniah, and Pethahiah, said, Stand up and bless the LORD your God forever and ever: and blessed be thy glorious name, which is exalted above all blessing and praise " (Nehemiah 9:5).

**Thy kingdom come.**

"And then shall appear the sign of the Son of man in heaven: and then shall all the tribes of the earth mourn, and they shall see the Son of man coming in the clouds of heaven with power and great glory" (Matthew 24:30).

**Thy will be done in earth,**

"For it is God which worketh in you both to will and to do of his good pleasure" (Philippians 2:13).

**As it is in heaven.**
"For I came down from heaven, not to do mine own will, but the will of him that sent me. And this is the Father's will which hath sent me, that of all which he hath given me I should lose nothing, but should raise it up again at the last day. And this is the will of him that sent me, that every one which seeth the Son, and believeth on him, may have everlasting life: and I will raise him up at the last day" (John 6:38-40).

**Give us this day our daily bread**.

"I am the LORD thy God, which brought thee out of the land of Egypt: open thy mouth wide, and I will fill it" (Psalms 81:10).

**And forgive us our debts**,

"Who is a God like unto thee, that pardoneth iniquity, and passeth by the transgression of the remnant of his heritage? He retaineth not his anger for ever, because he delighteth in mercy. He will turn again, he will have compassion upon us; he will subdue our iniquities; and thou wilt cast all their sins into the depths of the sea" (Micah 7:18, 19).

**As we forgive our debtors**.

"Then came Peter to him, and said, Lord, how oft shall my brother sin against me, and I forgive him? till seven times? Jesus saith unto him, I say not unto thee, Until seven times: but, Until seventy times seven " (Matthew 18:21, 22).

**And lead us not into temptation,**

"Let no man say when he is tempted, I am tempted of God: for God cannot be tempted with evil, neither tempteth he any man: But every man is tempted, when he is drawn away of his own lust, and enticed. Then when lust hath conceived, it bringeth forth sin: and sin, when it is finished, bringeth forth death" (James 1:13-15).

**But deliver us from evil:**

"Do ye think that the scripture saith in vain, The spirit that dwelleth in us lusteth to envy? But he giveth more grace. Wherefore he saith, God resisteth the proud, but giveth grace unto the humble. Submit yourselves therefore to God. Resist the devil, and he will flee from you. Draw nigh to God, and he will draw nigh to you. Cleanse your hands, ye sinners; and purify your hearts, ye double minded " (James 4:5-8).

**For thine is the kingdom,**

"All the ends of the world shall remember and turn unto the LORD: and all the kindreds of the nations shall worship before thee. For the kingdom is the LORD'S: and he is the governor among the nations. All they that be fat upon earth shall eat and worship: all they that go down to the dust shall bow before him: and none can keep alive his own soul" (Psalms 22:27-29).

61

## And the power,

"Trust not in oppression, and become not vain in robbery: if riches increase, set not your heart upon them. God hath spoken once; twice have I heard this; that power belongeth unto God" (Psalms 62:10,11).

## And the glory

"Then a cloud covered the tent of the congregation, and the glory of the LORD filled the tabernacle. And Moses was not able to enter into the tent of the congregation, because the cloud abode thereon, and the glory of the LORD filled the tabernacle. And when the cloud was taken up from over the tabernacle, the children of Israel went onward in all their journeys: But if the cloud were not taken up, then they journeyed not till the day that it was taken up" (Exodus 40:34-37).

## For ever.

"And I will betroth thee unto me for ever; yea, I will betroth thee unto me in righteousness, and in judgment, and in lovingkindness, and in mercies. I will even betroth thee unto me in faithfulness: and thou shalt know the LORD" (Hosea 2:19, 20).

## Amen.

"For all the promises of God in him are yea, and in him Amen, unto the glory of God by us" (2 Corinthians 1:20).
"And unto the angel of the church of the Laodiceans write; These things saith the Amen, the faithful and true witness, the beginning of the creation of God" (Revelation 3:14).
"He which testifieth these things saith, Surely I come quickly. Amen. Even so, come, Lord Jesus" (Revelation 22:20).

# Healing I

*Upon hearing about my diagnosis of prostate cancer, a member of my local church gave me the following list of Bible verses. She instructed me to read them regularly and to claim the miracle of healing from the Lord as He promised. I added a few of my favorite texts and appealed to God as family and friends prayed too. I thanked Him for His abundant blessings in the past, and I acknowledged His intervention in my life beyond my wildest dreams. For the present, I asked for God's guidance of the medical team that would attend to me. Even if I did not survive, I had already been blessed by His Providence from my youth. Praise God! I lived to tell the story.*

"Surely he hath borne our griefs, and carried our sorrows: yet we did esteem him stricken, smitten of God, and afflicted" (Isaiah 53:4).

"But he was wounded for our transgressions, he was bruised for our iniquities: the chastisement of our peace was upon him; and with his stripes we are healed" (Isaiah 53:5).

"Who his own self bare our sins in his own body on the tree, that we, being dead to sins, should live unto righteousness: by whose stripes we are healed" (1 Peter 2:24).

"And Jesus said unto the centurion, Go thy way; and as thou hast believed, so be it done unto thee. And his servant was healed in the selfsame hour.
And when Jesus was come into Peter's house, he saw his wife's mother laid, and sick of a fever.
And he touched her hand, and the fever left her: and she arose, and ministered unto them.
When the even was come, they brought unto him many that were possessed with devils: and he cast out the spirits with his word, and healed all that were sick:
That it might be fulfilled which was spoken by Esaias the prophet, saying, Himself took on our infirmities, and bare our sicknesses" (Matthew 8:13-17).

"Beloved, I wish above all things that thou mayest prosper and be in health, even as thy soul prospereth" (3 John 2).

"Is any among you afflicted? Let him pray. Is any merry? Let him sing psalms.
Is any sick among you? Let him call for the elders of the church; and let them pray over him, anointing him with oil in the name of the Lord:
And the prayer of faith shall save the sick, and the Lord shall raise him up; and if he have committed sins, they shall be forgiven him.

Confess your faults one to another, and pray one for another, that ye may be healed. The effectual fervent prayer of a righteous man availeth much" (James 5:13-17).

"And said, if thou wilt diligently harken to the voice of the Lord thy God, and wilt do that which is right in his sight, and wilt give ear to his commandments, and keep all his statutes, I will put none of these diseases upon thee, which I have brought upon the Egyptians: for I am the Lord that healeth thee" (Exodus 15:26).

"If my people, which are called by my name, shall humble themselves, and pray, and seek my face, and turn from their wicked ways; then I will hear from heaven, and will forgive their sin, and will heal their land" (2 Chronicles 7:14).

"For God hath not given us the spirit of fear; but of power, and of love, and of a sound mind" (2 Timothy 1:7).

"But we have this treasure in earthen vessels, that the excellency of the power may be of God, and not of us. We are troubled on every side, yet not distressed; we are perplexed, but not in despair; Persecuted, but not forsaken, cast down, but not destroyed " (2 Corinthians 4: 7-9).

# Open

A Meditation on Psalms 81:10, NKJV.

*"I am the Lord your God, which brought you out of the land of Egypt; Open your mouth wide, and I will fill it" (Psalm 81:10).*

The Speaker identifies Himself. He gives a specific example to bring the relationship into focus. He cites a well-known historic event. He gives His name and says what He did. With a reputation like that, God can speak with authority in order to command attention. The invitation continues....

## OPEN

Depending on God's intent, OPEN may be a command, a suggestion, a recommendation, an entreaty, or perhaps an invitation. At any rate, an action or a response is expected. At this point, the extent of the response isn't indicated. That's left to the discretion of the listener. But what's to be opened? Is this call a spiritual one, a physical one, or an emotional one? All of the above!

Am I an open person or a closed one? If I am open, I am receptive but vulnerable. If I am closed, I am deprived but protected. But am I open or closed to whom or to what? Does the choice have to be all or none? At the halfway mark, a container may be half empty or it may be half full. Here God says to open. I take Him at His word. I'm ready for further instructions.

## YOUR

The communication is now direct. True, YOUR may be plural. It could be singular. However, even if the remarks are directed to a group, singular responses are necessary. God doesn't mind relating one on one. So, I interpret that the invitation (command, recommendation, entreaty, suggestion) is for me. It's personal! I will use a mirror to focus the attention on my response. I will resist the urge to look around with a magnifying glass while checking to find out what others are doing: well, at least, on this occasion.

## MOUTH

The channel is identified. My MOUTH is a point of entry for nutrition. It's also a point of exit for words, or to spew out what is toxic. Consider the mouth to be symbolic. Then it could represent what I listen to, what I read, or what I understand. It could also be my attitude. And how about what I say, what I do, or what I think?

And how about my influence? This exercise is becoming quite personal. But that is what meditation is all about. Since I'm asking God to reveal Himself to me through this meditation, I'm going to listen and share what He reveals.

## WIDE

Although the choice is mine, this dimension is limitless. How wide is WIDE? It is up to me to take God at his word. He has a reputation of always coming through on His promises. So I may open my mouth as in a whisper and end up starving or at best undernourished. Or I may respond as though an examiner wants to see the back of my throat. But I'm usually a middle-of-the-road person. Therefore, I'll take in enough of what He offers to keep me in His good graces. Hold it! God might be encouraging me to stop holding back: to stop shortening His hands. After all, He did not hold back when He saved my life (seven times that I could recall).

## AND

This connecting word, AND, introduces the idea that something's about to be added: that is, if I should do my part. Again, the miserliness or the extravagance is mine to receive. It seems as though I must act according to by belief. At any rate, I've learned to trust in God: and I know that when He promises He delivers. It looks like He wants to come through for me again.

## I

The "I" refers to God. He already identified Himself as the One who started to speak.
It was He who delivered Israel from and slavery in Egypt.
It was He who sustained them in the wilderness.
It was He who was with them in later years.
He freed me from slavery to sin.
He sustains me daily.
He will be with me in the future.
So He is the One who is continuing to speak. This is not a directive from David, Asaph, Moses, Solomon, Ezra, or some other psalmist. I am boldly taking this invitation as coming from God to me.

## WILL

The promise is made. WILL means that what is promised is as good as delivered. I have tasted and seen that the Lord is good. I have asked, sought and found. I have knocked and doors have opened. With me, God has a reliable track record. Any time I doubt, all I have to do is to review how He has carried me on eagle's wings. He has come through for me in tangible ways–physically, emotionally, and spiritually. One translation states that God said that it was He who even opened the mouths of the Israelites.

## FILL

I just heard a song that says, "We are drinking from the saucer because the cup has overflowed." What a generous being God is! If I don't use what God provides, He only has to fill me once. But when I keep on using what He gives, when I share His blessings with others, when it takes His grace to help me through each day, I have to return to Him for refills. Imagine the God of the universe taking time to pay special attention to me! That is a very sobering thought. Sin has greatly reduced the efficiency of the human body. So God has to use high octane, engine cleaning, environment-friendly fuel to keep me going. God's grace is sufficient for me. FILL means that He does not do anything half way. I will never be empty except by my choice.

## IT

In the Gestalt concept of looking at experiences, the therapist invites the participant to use the first person pronoun in place of the word "IT." When I apply this method to this invitation, I can then say that God will fill me. Indeed, He has, and He continues to do so.

Infants frequently refuse to open their mouths when it is feeding time. They want to do something else. They simply will not open their mouths even after much coaxing. Finally we play the "garage and car game." They would rather play, so they open their mouths and we can then feed them. We get them to cooperate when we communicate in a language they understand. So it is with God. He constantly tries to find ways to reach us.

A personalized translation of the text might read as follows:
"I AM THE LORD, GOD, WHO BROUGHT RUDY FROM LA BREA, TRINIDAD, WEST INDIES, TO TUSCALOOSA, ALABAMA, USA. HE OPENED HIS HEART WIDE TO ME, AND I WILL CONTINUE TO FILL HIM BEYOND MEASURE." How about you? That's how it is with God! He meets us where we are in order to provide for us.

# Listen To Me

*At one of the most critical moments in Jesus' life, He called out to His Father addressing Him in an unusual manner. He repeated the name: Eloi, Eloi. It was as if His future depended on that decisive contact. Indeed, it did. He had to be sure that His agonizing plea got through. Jesus had used that same type of salutation before. That was how he addressed Martha and Simon Peter. On the Damascus road, Saul heard his name repeated and he knew that it was Jesus who called. This style, name repetition, identifies Jesus as the Caller who spoke to Abraham, Jacob, Moses, and little Samuel in Old Testament times.*

### Abraham

"And the angel of the LORD called unto him out of heaven, and said, **Abraham, Abraham**: and he said, Here am I. And he said, Lay not thine hand upon the lad, neither do thou any thing unto him: for now I know that thou fearest God, seeing thou hast not withheld thy son, thine only son from me" (Genesis 22:11,12).

### Jacob

"And Israel took his journey with all that he had, and came to Beersheba, and offered sacrifices unto the God of his father Isaac. And God spake unto Israel in the visions of the night, and said, **Jacob, Jacob**. And he said, Here am I. And he said, I am God, the God of thy father: fear not to go down into Egypt; for I will there make of thee a great nation: I will go down with thee into Egypt; and I will also surely bring thee up again: and Joseph shall put his hand upon thine eyes" (Genesis 46:1-4).

### Moses

"And the angel of the LORD appeared unto him in a flame of fire out of the midst of a bush: and he looked, and, behold, the bush burned with fire, and the bush was not consumed. And Moses said, I will now turn aside, and see this great sight, why the bush is not burnt. And when the LORD saw that he turned aside to see, God called unto him out of the midst of the bush, and said, **Moses, Moses**. And he said, Here am I. And he said, Draw not nigh hither: put off thy shoes from off thy feet, for the place whereon thou standest is holy ground " (Exodus 3:2-5).

## Samuel

"And the LORD called Samuel again the third time. And he arose and went to Eli, and said, Here am I; for thou didst call me. And Eli perceived that the LORD had called the child. Therefore Eli said unto Samuel, Go, lie down: and it shall be, if he call thee, that thou shalt say, Speak, LORD; for thy servant heareth. So Samuel went and lay down in his place. And the LORD came, and stood, and called as at other times, **Samuel, Samuel.** Then Samuel answered, Speak; for thy servant heareth" (1 Samuel 3:8-10).

## Martha

"And Jesus answered and said unto her, **Martha, Martha**, thou art careful and troubled about many things. But one thing is needful: and Mary hath chosen that good part, which shall not be taken away from her" (Luke10: 41, 42).

## Simon Peter

"And the Lord said, **Simon, Simon**, behold, Satan hath desired to have you, that he may sift you as wheat: But I have prayed for thee, that thy faith fail not: and when thou art converted, strengthen thy brethren" (Luke 22:31, 32).

## Eloi

"And at the ninth hour Jesus cried with a loud voice, saying, **Eloi, Eloi**, lama sabachthani? which is, being interpreted, My God, my God, why hast thou forsaken me?" (Mark 15:34).

## Saul

"And as he journeyed, he came near Damascus: and suddenly there shined round about him a light from heaven: And he fell to the earth, and heard a voice saying unto him, **Saul, Saul**, why persecutest thou me? And he said, Who art thou, Lord? And the Lord said, I am Jesus whom thou persecutest: it is hard for thee to kick against the pricks. And he trembling and astonished said, Lord, what wilt thou have me to do? And the Lord said unto him, Arise, and go into the city, and it shall be told thee what thou must do" (Acts 9:3-6).

———◆◆◆———

**It is what happens after the wake-up call that determines its outcome.**

———◆◆◆———

# Pathways to Success

*This item is an expansion of a concept I wrote about in "Building A Sound Mind," Message Magazine, Vol. 58, No. 3 May/June 1992.*

*Many circumstances helped to shape my life. Out of them I developed these guidelines for success. I originally came across some of these items in a table tennis magazine. Over the years I modified the items as they applied to me, and I added Biblical support for the steps.*

*As with any developmental scheme, there is a sense of progression. However, the stages are not discrete entities: there is overlap; there are periods of returning to earlier ones; there are times of jumping ahead. Nevertheless, the outline serves me well. It may also be converted into a grid with the seven pathways as rows and the columns divided into time lines (days, months, quarters, years, etc.). In that case a separate chart may be used for each plan or project.*

1.  PAUSE. Slow down. Take an inventory of your life. When you want to set your sight on goals, you have to stop before you start. It's like taking an inventory. One Old Testament prophet said, "Consider your ways" (Haggai 1:5).

2.  PRAY. Praying is recognizing the importance and influence of the Creator of the universe in your life. After all, He brought you into existence. Calling on Him and listening to His response allows you to discover your purpose here. God has not left you to manage life's experiences by yourself. "Trust in the Lord with all thine heart; and lean not unto thine own understanding. In all thy ways acknowledge him, and he shall direct thy paths" (Proverbs 3:5,6). Praying includes more than asking for direction. It also means praising Him. Follow the example of the lone leper who returned to say thanks to Jesus for being healed as described in Luke 17:17.

3.   PLAN. Set goals and seek counsel about them. Make room for periodic adjustments. At an early age, Jesus was aware that His life had a special purpose. He asked His parents if they did not know that He had to be about His Father's business (Luke 2:49). Adults may ask for direction, too. The Apostle Paul did so when he said, "Lord, what will thou have me to do?" (Acts 9:6). In the process you will have to adjust your priorities. You will come to some tough choices just as the decision that the young man faced when Jesus asked him to sell all that he had (Matthew 19:21).

4.   PRINCIPLES. Instead of depending on assumptions, learn the rules, regulations and expectations of your goals or projects. Inquire about how to get to where you want to go. Seek counsel. The laws of nature, health, relationships, the community, work, academics, etc., apply to all situations except when God chooses to step in with a miracle. Be prepared to meet the requirements. The Bible says of Ezra that he was a "ready scribe" (Ezra 7:6). He really knew his craft.

5.   PRACTICE. Noble intentions are of no value unless you put them into action. If you want your dream to come true, you have to wake up and do your part. If you open your mouth, God will fill it as He promised (Psalms 81:10). Be careful what you practice, though, because you will become good at it, whether the habit is good or bad.

6.   PERSEVERE. You will inevitably meet obstacles. When you decide to work toward a goal, you will meet distractions. If you expect consistent results too early, you invite frustration. You will have to give up your membership in the procrastinators club. You will have to continue on your new course relentlessly. Focus. The hardship you will encounter is the price you pay for not going along aimlessly with the crowd. In John 17:15 Jesus prayed that His disciples would be protected in their hardships rather than spared from them.

7.   PROMOTE. Now it is your turn to share. Other people have encouraged you along the way and have contributed to your success. You are a collage of your past. Now you may encourage others. God has placed you amidst people just when you had one kind of need or another. So, allow yourself to be a guide to someone else. The Samaritan woman who met Jesus at the well was so enthusiastic about her new discovery that she had to pass it on (John 4:28, 29).

———◆———

| | |
|---|---|
| **In a toxic conversation you may have to LURD:** | **Listen,** |
| | **Understand,** |
| | **Repeat,** |
| | **Disengage.** |
| | |
| **But in a nutritious one you LURE:** | **Listen,** |
| | **Understand,** |
| | **Repeat,** |
| | **Engage.** |

———◆———

# The Two Camps of Change

*Our efforts to adjust to the constantly changing environment often place us into one of two general categories: for or against. So we belong to one of two camps. Our actions indicate where we fit.*

*The Order of the Eternal Optimists*

Channel your energies.
Huddle with motivated people.
Anticipate obstacles and work around them.
Neutralize the negatives.
Generate enthusiasm.
Expect positive results.

*The Association Against Anything*

Complain every chance you get.
Honor the codes of the status quo.
Antagonize, aggravate, and agitate.
Negate any evidence of improvement.
Gang up against anyone who tries to improve things.
Enjoy the benefits of the very changes you oppose.

**Two friends wanted what was best, but one went east, and the other went west.**

———◆◆◆———

# Chips From The Sculptor's Chisel

The experiences of life:
    God's methods of getting our attention
        and reshaping us into His image.
           A sculptor hacks, gouges, rasps, drills, veneers,
                bends, chisels, molds, sands,
                    and polishes raw material
                        to produce a priceless work of art.
Similarly,
    challenges of life
        provide various opportunities
           for refinement.

Endure the process.

Hacking is like changing *impulsiveness* into *patience*,
           *Vindictiveness* into *forgiveness*,
             *Selfishness* into *benevolence*,
              *Vulgarity* into *refinement*.

Gouging is like reshaping *haste* into *composure*,
           *Unconcern* into *love*,
             *Isolation* into *involvement*,
             *Bias* into *tolerance*.

Rasping is like transforming *quandary* into *quietude*,
           *Insecurity* into *confidence*,
             *Guilt* into *innocence*,
             *Disturbance* into *peace*.

Drilling is like altering *neglect* into *validation,*
    *Blindness* into *sight,*
    *Control* into *cooperation,*
    *Selfishness* into *benevolence.*

Veneering is like redesigning *suspicions* into *trust,*
    *Delusions* into *reality,*
    *Anger* into *tolerance,*
    *Forgetfulness* into *recall.*

Bending is like converting *self-centeredness* into *gratitude,*
    *Doubt* into *assurance,*
    *Dread* into *bravery,*
    *Folly* into *wisdom.*

Chiseling is like remodeling *obstinacy* into *submission,*
    *Disarray* into *order,*
    *Pride* into *humility,*
    *Silence* into *expression.*

Molding is like recasting *weeping* into *joy,*
    *Barrenness* into *fertility,*
    *Hesitancy* into *eagerness,*
    *Bondage* into *freedom.*

Sanding is like altering *arrogance* into *meekness,*
    *Sickness* into *health,*
    *Pain* into *relief,*
    *Tiredness* into *rest.*

Polishing is like refining *discouragement* into *hope,*
    *Distraction* into *focus,*
    *Mediocrity* into *excellence,*
    *Failure* into *progress.*

Enjoy the result.

# Acceptance

*During the funeral service for one of my goddaughters who died in an automobile accident six weeks after my surgery, the weeping congregation wrestled silently with the loss. She had shown such promise! The presiding minister approached the rostrum to invite God's continued presence, but he, too, tried in vain to stop his flow of tears. Speaking between sobs, he began the eulogy. Just then, with words which could only come in answer to our collective prayer he said, "What we cannot now understand, we must accept." I interrupted my grief long enough to write down some seed thoughts on those comforting words and completed the composition upon my return home.*

**ALTER** your preconceived notion of what has happened by replacing it with what the Bible says about such calamities.

**CONSIDER** that while you may know a lot there's still more for you to learn about illness, death, disappointment, or any other type of trauma, especially when it comes without warning.

**CONFER** with others who have wrestled successfully with similar issues. Draw on their strength.

**EXERCISE** the faith you've been developing in your walk with God. It just might be that you were being prepared for times like these.

**PAUSE** once in a while. Excessive rumination on the same challenge can lead to mental, physical, and spiritual exhaustion. So take a break. Rest in the Lord.

**TELL** yourself that others have successfully come to grips with death and loss, and that you will also.

**ANALYZE** your progress and be thankful for where you are now. Remember, you are not alone.

**NEUTRALIZE** the sorrow, sadness, and despondency that accompany the loss by remembering the pleasant and joyful times you had with the deceased loved one.

**CONFESS** any sins or misgivings. They may be holding you back and depriving you of the very relief you seek.

**ENJOY** the peace that comes even in sorrow.

---

**I may not like it when you are right and I am wrong, but I surely do like the benefits.**

---

# Alphabet Soup for Couples

ANNIVERSARIES. That yearly number that husbands can't seem to be able to remember. But wives do.

BIRTHDAYS. The dates that come around too slowly when you are young and too quickly when you are old.

CHILDBEARING.  The process our wives wish we would try–just once.

DEAR.  The over emphasized pet name that husbands use when we are angry at our wives and we try to hide it.

EXPECTATION. Wanting our wives to read our minds without coming out and saying so.

FORGIVENESS.  The gift we are eager to receive but reluctant to give.

GENEROSITY.  Giving without wanting anything back–but taking it anyway.

HOME.  The place you just can't wait to get to only to find out that it is just like what you ran from.

INTIMACY. Repeated and purposeful occupation of each other's spiritual, mental, and physical space.

JUNK. The precious works of art that the other spouse calls worthless.

KISSING. An oral habit we learned in childhood that we keep on practicing way into adulthood.

LOTION. The liquid a wife wishes her husband would discover before he puts his hands on her.

MEMORIES. The events a husband and a wife remember so differently that we wonder if we were both there at the same time.

NAGGING. When the wife is asking the tenth question while the husband is still trying to figure out the first answer.

OPINIONS. The safe answers we make up instead of admitting that we don't know.

PARADISE. The place we went on our wedding day and to which we spend the rest of our life trying to return.

QUESTION. That is something we want to ask (but we are afraid to) when our spouse insists that we do something the way her parent did it, and we want to know why she did not marry that parent.

REASSURANCE. That is what we need when our get-up-and-go got-up-and-left, but we don't want to believe it.

SILENCE. The safety zone that helps us to buy some time when we don't know what to do next.

TACKY. That's how we look when we think our colors match.

UNDERESTIMATE. That's what happens to a two-hundred-pound husband when he realizes that his one-hundred-pound wife disagrees with him and she's not about to back down.

VULNERABLE. Waiting for comments when we undress before each other for the first time—and we are not sure why the other person is not saying anything—just staring.

WISDOM. Knowing when the truth about certain sensitive subjects is not what the other person really wants to hear at that time.

X-RAY VISION. The uncanny ability wives possess, which allows them to see through husbands without the aid of any special equipment.

YIELD. That's what we should do when we put our foot in our mouth and the more we try to take it out the worse it gets.

ZANY. That is what this ALPHABET SOUP is all about.

---

**You are a disarmingly humble gentleman...(but you just won't fit in with us).**

---

# Black History Alphabet

Advancement.
Build bridges instead of walls.
Connect with people with similar interests.
Discovering your place in the struggle.
Expect improvement.
Forgive.
Growing in grace.
Heal–emotionally, racially, and spiritually.
Inspire the youth.
Joining hands.
Kneel to ask God for strength to carry on.
Love especially when it is hard to do.
Mend relationships.
Neutralize negative influences.
Opportunities come. Look for them.
Praise God for not forgetting us.
Question inequity.
Remember where you came from.
Share experiences to encourage others.
Tame anger and redirect energy.
Understand differences.
Vote for change.
Working together.
[E]Xamine your motives.
Yearn for better days.
Zeal sometimes requires balance.

**If you need me just call… (but it doesn't mean that I'll come).**

---

# Control

(The other side of insecurity)

COMPETE rather than cooperate.

ORDER instead of ask or negotiate.

NEGATIVE statements and put-downs abound.

THREATENING language and attitude reign.

RULERSHIP instead of partnership is the style. The adage, "give and take" is interpreted as "I give and you take."

OPTIONS are not encouraged.

LOYALTY is expected at all cost.

---

**"What wake-up call? Are you kidding? I haven't even gone to bed as yet."**

---

# Disability

**D** YSFUNCTION occurs in areas of your body that adversely affect both your ability to work and your self-image.

**I** NVENTORY your past levels of performance in comparison with current limitations and future challenges.

**S** ELFCONSCIOUSNESS of your condition is a frequent mental intruder and distracter.

**A** NXIETY about your ability and capacity to adjust is a major reality.

**B** ENEFITS to be received financially may or may not be sufficient to allow the future quality of life for which you were planning upon retirement.

**I** NITIATIVE is needed in order to revive past hobbies, develop new interests, or continue current ones.

**L** ONGING for the good old days is common. This state of mind, if allowed to persist, will rob you of time and energy that can be put to good use.

**I** NSPIRATION from your support system of family and friends is an antidote for discouragement.

**T** ALK to others who are in a similar situation although they may not share much.

**Y** IELDING to negative or to positive influences determines your outcome.

# Diversity

Celebrate the **D**IGNITY of human life.

Know that **I**NTERDEPENDENCE is a double blessing.

Appreciate the **V**ALUE of a different opinion.

You are an **E**XAMPLE.

**R**ESPECT your uniqueness.

**S**HARE the earth.

Do not be afraid to **I**NITIATE dialogue.

Regain lost **T**RUST.

Make efforts to heal **Y**ESTERDAY'S wounds.

———◆—◆———

**You do not have to accept or even believe what you are expected to know if you want to join certain special interest groups. Just repeat it to the satisfaction of the keeper of the gate whose domain you desire to enter.**

———◆—◆———

# Frustration

**F** EELING apprehensive when expectations are not met.

**R** EGRESSING to an earlier stage of life with pouting and wanting immediate relief.

**U** RGENTLY demanding immediate relief in the absence of a real crisis.

**S** ULKING that continues with endless questions and requests for relief.

**T** EMERITY. How can anyone dare to make me wait?

**R** EGRETS come to mind when choices cannot be reversed.

**A** NGER, poorly focused, that feeds on itself.

**T** OMORROW may never come, it seems.

**9** NSECURITY. IMPATIENCE. IRRITABLENESS.

**0** UTRAGEOUS behavior that is humorous by hindsight.

**N** OTHING seems to satisfy.

# Healing II

**H** ARNESS the best available remedies for your illness. Look at the various options before you make your decision.

**E** DUCATE yourself about your condition.

**A** VOID negative influences when you recognize them.

**L** AUNCH a program of lifestyle change to continue the healing process.

**I** NSPIRE others to pay attention to, and to act on, warning signals.

**N** URTURE yourself physically, mentally, and spiritually.

**G** OD will see you through.

---

**" Please (yawn), you have the wrong room (yawn) again; I didn't (yawn) ask for a wake-up call. Is this (yawn) April Fool?"**

---

# Patience

**P** ONDER the possibility of choosing other options.

**A** SSESS the value of what you desire.

**T** RUST that you will receive what you need on time. (Send some one to the nursing station.)

**I** NVITE an atmosphere of peace.

**E** NTERTAIN the notion that responses come in the form of "yes," "wait," "perhaps," or "no."

**N** EGATE the toxic thoughts, feelings, and actions you experience.

**C** ONSIDER that you are a part of the universe, but you are not the center.

**E** NDURE the process now without making it worse so that you may ENJOY the results later.

———————◆————————

**I'll keep you in my prayers… (I can talk to God, but I can't talk to you).**

———————◆————————

# Prayer

**P** OUR out your heart to God without reservation.

**R** EAD God's Word to grasp how He has dealt with others in similar situations and to discover what He wants to say to you.

**A** CCEPT what God reveals to you.

**Y** EARN to be close to God without avoidance of close personal relationships.

**E** XERCISE implicit faith.

**R** EJOICE in the assurance that the God of the universe takes time to commune with you.

---

**Who'd have thought that you'd get this far...?**
**(I really didn't think you had it in you).**

# Recovery

**R** ELIEF, at least partially, from many of the restrictions and limitations I thought would never go away.

**E** XPECTING that I would adjust although I couldn't quite see it as yet.

**C** OUNTING my blessings: Not just taking them for granted.

**O** PTIMISM about my lot helped to hasten the healing process: the Bible says it and science agrees.

**U** ALUING the support of family and friends who stuck by me even when I tried to shut them out during my periods of self-pity.

**E** XERCISING my body, mind, and spirit even when I didn't feel like it. Positive results followed.

**R** EJOICING that although I was not where I wanted to be in my progress, I was no longer where I used to be.

**Y** ESTERDAY'S dreams had to be modified: but I continued to dream anyway.

---

# Mysteries

*I scrutinized scraps of wood from a broken directors chair. Out of the heap I salvaged a few pieces and transformed them into a toy house with furniture.*

So it was through
                    Mending
                        Yielding
                            Surviving
                                Triumphing
                                    Enduring
                                Recovering
                            Improving
                        Emancipating
                    Struggling
                        that the Master Carpenter mended my broken life.

# Suppose

Suppose black meant white and up meant down,
Then day would be night and a smile would be a frown.
Suppose ugly meant pretty and wet meant dry,
Then sane would be nutty and shut would be pry.

Suppose a feast meant a famine and stop meant go.
Then ignore would be examine and yes would mean no.
Suppose hide meant show and smaller meant larger,
Then ebb would be flow and now would be later.

Suppose nadir meant zenith and in meant out,
Then skin would be pith and settle would be scout.
Suppose pleasure meant pain and bitter meant sweet,
Then loss would mean gain and starve would mean treat.

Suppose wise meant foolish and cut meant mend,
Then mature would mean young and start would mean end.
Suppose rend meant join and smooth meant rough,
Then doubt would mean believe and tender would mean tough.

Suppose tall meant short and full meant empty,
Then sold would mean bought and dearth would mean plenty.
Suppose left meant right and low meant high.
Then dull would be witty and laugh would be cry.

But "break a leg" means good luck and "bad" clothes are good.
So, when I say, "I won't," do I mean I would?
And when I say, " I can't" do I mean I could?

# Picnic at Sycamore

Many were playing and having fun.
Some sat in the shade to avoid the sun.
I took out some paper to write the score
For the church picnic at Sycamore.

A toddler was pushing a red toy rig.
I stooped, but she said I was still too big.
She never gave poor, sad me a ride
To save my face I ran to the slide.

Just then a sister saw me writing.
She thought that I was just composing.
My attitude she misconstrued.
My mind was simply on the food.

As custom here down in the South,
We gathered in groups to run our mouth.
Men by themselves: The women too.
The latest private pots to stew.

I felt so young I played some ball.
I ran so hard I thought I'd fall.
I pulled a muscle I forgot I had–
For the next few days I hurt real bad.

The picnic came off very well.
By the look on our faces I could tell.
We finally followed Jesus' style,
"Come ye apart and rest awhile."

All those whose names I did not mention,
Alas,  dear hearts, it was my intension
To leave you out so you would pout
And give me something to write about.

# Sycamore Afterthought

The sycamore poem seemed a bit short.
"More things to say," I bet you thought.
I did not mean to burst your bubble;
I left out your name, now I'm in trouble.

One person described as very nice
This day didn't bring the usual ice.
No one told me, but I did overhear
The melon came from a sister dear.

Brother A brought this, and sister B did that.
Without each one, it would have fallen flat.
I know your name you wanted to see.
Dig deep down inside–have mercy on me.

89

"Operator, what happened to my wake-up call?" "Sir, our record shows that
we gave it two hours ago."

———◆———

# A Psalm of the Prostate

The prostate is my shepherd. I lack nothing.

It makes me lie down, and sleep peacefully. It leads me to the arms of my
mate.

It restores my status that I am the man.

It leads me in the paths of pleasantries and procreation for my own name's sake.

Yea, though I hear that thousands of men are diagnosed with prostate cancer
every year and that many of them will die from it, I will hide my symptoms such as
urinary frequency, hesitation, or even a speck of blood.

I will fear no prostate disease.

For my prostate will always be healthy. It will always be with me.

I cannot see it, but I know it is there. Along with related organs, it comforts me.

It allows me the delight of macho status even if that is vanity. It feeds my ego.

I am so satisfied I can hardly stand myself.

Surely, I thought that it would stay with me all the days of my life:

I refuse to think it would be gone, forever.

———◆———

# To Mother

I saw my mother work
From early morn 'till after set of sun.
I saw my mother sleep
After a heavy task
Accomplished, done.

I saw my mother pray
For strength to live the life she had begun.
I saw my mother shine
With light
Reflecting
From the Golden Sun.

I saw my mother lean
On kitchen sink to prop herself with love.
I glimpsed my mother's pain
Concealed.
Her strength
Came from above.

I saw my mother end
The race she ran with pride.
And on the floor her lifeless posture said,
"Please let them know,
My son,
I tried."

**When I see you, I don't see you as being Black…**
**(I don't want to deal with what your blackness evokes in me).**

# Invisibility

I am silent.
But that does not mean I cannot speak.
Because I do not speak,
That does not mean I have nothing to say.
Please notice me!

My eyes are closed.
But that does not mean I cannot see.
Because I do not see,
That does not mean I'm not informed.
Please notice me!

I do not mix.
But that does not mean I am aloof.
Because I do not move,
That does not mean I want to be alone.
Please notice me!

I do not sing.
But that does not mean I cannot sing.
Because I do not sing,
That does not mean I do not know the song.
Please notice me!

My skin is not like yours.
But that does not mean we are so different.
Because we're not alike,
That does not mean we can't relate.
Hello!

**It is less threatening to use a magnifying glass to examine a situation in order to blame the other person than it is to use a mirror to discover your part of the problem.**

# The Mold

Dare to talk to me about me!
I am different from the rest.

Talk about others you know.
Exclude no gender.

OK! Write
From the pages of your memory
How she always "told" him but did not "ask" him.
How nothing was ever in the place where she left it.
And the furniture had to be moved, again.
Or the things he did: like leaving clothes where he undressed,
Or forgetting promises, birthdays, or anniversaries,
And avoiding cut flowers because they die quickly.

Go ahead! Disguise
Place of residence, name, gender,
Stranger, spouse, or vocation.
Hide the identity of friend, kin, or offspring.
Yet, no mirror could contrive such diversity of roles.

Enough!
Now let me add one more for him:
Consider the safe retreat of silence.
And for her:
Infractions long since committed return as new.

Ah! Table of Contents!
Regardless of the story told,
It seemed you called my name.
There is a mold!

# Where Did You Go?

We spoke.
The subject seemed interesting.
I heard what you said
Before you changed your voice.
You changed your face too.

I waited.
You spoke but made no sound.
You looked right through me
Without a blink.

You left although you did not move.
Your brain flashed
Pictures I could not see.
Where did you go?

# Thin Skin

Don't come to church if your skin is thin.
Something might happen to you within.
Someone might make you slip and sin.
You might even see your twin.

Don't come to church if your skin is thin.
A member might try your soul to win.
A new life surely you will begin.
Remember the church is anti-sin.

Don't come to church if your skin is thin.
The smile you see might just be a grin.
Your balloons might burst to your chagrin
If you get close to the Gospel pin.

Well, come to church though your skin is thin.
Listen above the confusing din.
We know, for all of us have been
Plagued by the turmoil and pickle you're in.

# Bring Back the Welcome Mat

I come to worship God
And fellowship with you,
But things get turned around.
I don't know what to do.

The Good Book says to meet
With folks like you and pray.
I come and find a cozy seat
And then you move away.

I meditate and thank
Him for His only Son.
But when I reach across the pew
My company you shun.

I dare not let you know
The hurt you cannot see.
I've carried it so long
It's like a part of me.

I came for strength that day.
You told me I would find
Forgiveness for my sins
And friends that're true and kind.

The words sound fine and sweet;
They're music to my ear.
But when I open up to you
You act like you don't care.

If Jesus cleaned you up
You'd know the way I feel.
Perhaps you're hurting, too–
It does take time to heal.

If that's the case, dear friend,
I want something that's real.
On you I can't depend.
Where is the Christian zeal?

The heartaches that you bear
Leave little space for mine.
I thought you laid them down
When you believed the Vine.

It seems you cast them down
And forthwith picked them up.
So how can you reach me
And walk with a full cup?

I'd like to stay. I really would.
The message seemed quite clear.
I need relief today.
His coming seems so near.

So ask me back some time.
I pray that you would heed
The task that Jesus gave–
To guide some one in need.

# Helpless Not Hopeless

I am a hostage free
To do just as I please.
But all you do is pray
And stay down on your knees.

These stories that you tell
Show me I'm left behind.
There's nothing you can say
To make me change my mind.

These walls, they come and go
No matter where I am.
Okay, you told me so.
I should have listened, Mom.

The world owes me my keep.
My friends all tried and failed.
So even if you weep,
Just come and have me bailed.

I live like I don't care.
The old and new don't mix.
That slavery stuff's still there;
It's just a bag of tricks.

You say that things have changed,
God will this world remake.
But I am not deranged.
What difference will it make?

You always tried your best
The world to make me see.
I want to pass the test,
So don't give up on me.

# Don't Call Me

Don't call me a snob
Because I speak only to people I choose to,
Or do things,
Or go places I want to
And leave when I am ready.

Don't call me a snob
When I give a good tongue-lashing
To people who violate my personal space
Or disregard my unpublished rules.

Don't call me a snob
When acquaintances
Fail to see the world through my eyes
Or march to my beat.

Don't call me a snob
When I expect people to remember
What I say the first time. I don't like to
repeat myself.
In fact!

Just don't call me.

## Help Meet

One day we became one, you and I.
That day your eyes became mine.
Your ears became mine.
Your tongue became mine.
Your feet became mine.
Your brain became mine.

Then one day I could not see,
And I could not hear,
And I could not speak,
And I could not walk,
And I could not remember.

But we are still one, you and I.
So I can still see,
   Hear,
     Speak,
      Walk,
And I can still remember, through you.
For you are my HELP MEET.

## More Than

I am more than what I see.
I am more than what I hear.
I am more than what I touch.
I am more than what I taste.
I am more than what I smell.
I am more than what I think.
I am more than what I say.
I am more than what I learn.
I am more than what I produce.
I am more than what I eat.
I am more than what I drink.

When I became what I am,
I became more than what I was.
I lost! I gained!
So, now, instead of being less,
**I am MORE THAN–**

# O Precious Life, Now Shortened

*A commentary on the brief life of Elisa Roseann Moore, June 8, 1979 - November 7, 2000: It may be sung to the tune of the hymn, "O Sacred Head Now Wounded."*

What language shall I borrow to speak of you dear child?
Your life had shown such promise, your manner firm, yet mild.
Without your choice, dear traveler: yours, the immigrants' fate.
How did you keep old values and yet live up to date?

You looked up to your brother though junior, he, by far.
Molded by your dear mother you were a rising star.
Your love for your dear father shone through tenaciously.
Fam'ly with miles unnumbered preserved though scattered be.

The world became your backyard. Ambition knew no bound.
Your place in God's Work waiting, searching but not yet found.
While on your way to worship the God who saved your soul,
Your exit was so sudden. We know you reached your goal.

For those who have survived you: kinfolk or friend or foe,
Your passing is this lesson: One day each one must go.
The manner does not matter, for sin its course must run.
Live fully for the Savior. Expect to hear "Well Done."

Let no distraction, therefore, in thought or word or deed,
Entice us from His favor; our questions He will heed.
Our finite minds still groping for solace small or grand.
One day, with veil removed, all acts we'll understand.

And now a note from Auntie, who loved you as her own.
When months of absence passed by she'd say, "How well you've grown."
But now farewell, My Precious, we sing our parting song.
Sleep sweet 'till Jesus calls you; the wait will not be long.

**If you knew it was thought that what you did couldn't be done you wouldn't have done it.**

———◆———

# It Doesn't Cost. It Pays

You see me now and you assume
That you know me quite well.
You're dazzled by the place I room.
Let me my story tell.

You may be right, but just in part.
This mountain top you know.
So stop to ask, "Where did it start?"
A vale or two ago.

Please look beyond what you can see;
Some scars you just might find.
There really is much more to me.
Hold still while I unwind.

With youthful zest and vision bright
The way seemed very clear.
I'd press right on with all my might
But snags were in the air.

To learn a trade I had been sent.
My mother could not pay.
To lead, not follow, was my bent,
To earn, the only way.

While cars and trucks I did repair
And still a little green,
I rose in status 'twas quite clear,
Pushed by a Force unseen.

New machines came, out went the old.
An Englishman my guide.
A high promotion I could hold
If I would stem the tide.

He said at first, "The pipes we'll hit
With hammer to remove
The rust and dirt; each little bit
Could damage any groove."

We struck and struck. What noise we made!
And then he went away.
But soon returned in a tirade
That awful, dreadful day.

The noise came to a sudden end.
My buttocks he did kick.
An enemy! That was no friend.
It felt worse than a brick.

He looked at me. I looked at him.
We both in silence stood.
My future weighed in balance grim,
I could not see the good.

Now with the hammer in my hand
I quickly checked the range.
A fatal blow I sure could land
And my whole life would change.

I stood and looked up at his head
And then I saw his knees.
With just one blow he could be dead
And hush his useless pleas.

With youthful age and exercise
My biceps–they did bulge.
To show them off could win a prize
Oh yes! I did indulge.

99

But in a flash my life I saw
In very plain detail.
The sentence would be "life" by law.
One day I'd die in jail.

I dropped the hammer on the floor.
Just why? I had no clue.
Among my friends I knew I'd score.
But what would Jesus do?

God made me lay that hammer down,
And turn the other cheek.
So I would gain the golden crown
'Twas He who made me meek.

No college dream? No plans unfold?
No parent to repay?
All would be lost when story told
Of my response that day.

That kick, you see, was Satan's plan
To throw me off the track.
And emphasize the carnal man
With hateful striking back.

That day I earned the medal gold
For Best Apprenticeship.
It boosted me to heights untold
Because I did not slip.

Back to the plan to school I went,
Determined to fulfill
The early dreams by Jesus sent
And strengthened by His will.

So what you see around me here
May dazzle some, that's true.
A little glimpse I tried to share
Let God prove it to you.

I hide the hurt to carry on.
That helps in many ways.
And when I think of days now gone
It does not cost. It pays.

———◆———

**The desire to control another person is often a façade for insecurity.**

———◆———

100

# Abuseville

The City of Victims is a horrible place
Where people get started in a terrible race.
They did not ask to fall from grace
Whatever the speed, it's a tragic pace.

The City of Victims is easy to find.
Its people you spot if even you're blind.
Signs of hurt and a life in a bind
Like citrus leave a trail behind.

The City of Victims makes room for more,
Whose bodies still ache and hearts quite sore.
No need explain or give whole score;
The memories are vivid, the trauma still raw.

The City of Victims has streets of dope.
Some lives are wrecked; it appears no hope.
Your kind concern, what a rescue a rope!
Such heartfelt ways do help to cope.

The City of Victims respects no class.
Abuse of all kinds extends their morass.
Young, innocent, filled with trespass,
None are immune. There's no safety pass.

The City of Victims, like an endless spiral,
Puts whole world around you each day on trial.
The hurt constructs a wall of denial
Each passing day, a matter of survival.

———◆◆◆———

**I was just going to call you…(it is a good thing you called).**

———◆◆◆———

# The Meeting

The name is really quite absurd;
We ought to use a different word.
Instead of saying we had a meeting
Let's say instead we had a beating.

The leader asked a question clear;
One person tried to take the chair.
Another sulked at how things were going
'Twas then true colors started showing.

First one said this. Another said that.
Before we knew it we had a spat.
Our tongues clashed hard. Our heels did click.
I, myself, put in a lick.

At meetings we share and ideas exchange
In order to plan and good programs arrange.
At beatings the choice is easy to make.
It's my way or the highway take.

If you dare lead and plan a sitting,
Remember that this is not a meeting.
Be sure to come to dodge my arrow.
Forget about the straight and narrow.

You know I cannot end this way
The Word must have a bit to say.
When you sit down, my brethren dear,
Remember what you said in prayer.

All things conduct with decency.
Of envy, pride you must be free.
Each one preferring other more,
That way feelings can't end up sore.

The reason for the plans you lay
Apply to all of us. Each day,
Dear friends, do not behave unwise.
O shameful thought to miss the Prize!

# Sun Cycle

### Sunset

The orange globe no longer ablaze
Dipped behind the dark green shadowed trees
And ushered in a bright new day
Of golden opportunities.

### Midnight

Nothing in nature told me that you came.
Not brightness!
Not length of shadow!
Not beauty of changing colors!
I had to check the clock.
It whispered, "Twelve."

### Sunrise

You arrived at precise moment in my town
At first perceptible light,
At first burst of brightness,
At first peep over towering mountain,
At roosters' announcing crow and mockingbird's wakening song.
I could not tell which!
I only know you came.

### Midday

From the zenith of its daily celestial arc
The pulsating fiery orb
Aimed raging radiant rays
At earth,
Scarcely casting a soothing shadow.

Sunset

The thirsty, reddened brine slowly swallowed the sinking sun
Like a glazed donut center
Slipping reluctantly
From inexperienced dunking fingers.

---

**You're always on my mind...(no wonder I can't think clearly).**

---

# Truth Changed My Face

I reached for you.
My open hand changed into a fist:
Grasping nothing but air.

Months passed to years,
And love to endless hope.
Tears reddened my eyes.
Pain aged my cheeks.
Memories dimmed my charm.

Versions of truth fell from guessing lips.
Each well intended tale propelling one awful lack–
It did not bring you back.

My youthful frame
Could not withstand the strain.
We could not stay the same.

In silence now
Stand and stare!
Recall the year!
Find a trace!

The truth, yet untold.
But still it changed my face.

---

**If we would compete less and cooperate more we would become
an unbeatable team.**

---

# Last Words

As husband I thought I had the last word,
But soon found out that was absurd.
Our talks would often end in strife.
I dared out-talk my newfound wife.

For any marriage to survive
Two little words keep it alive.
It takes some time to see the light
Or things will end up in a fight.

Not openly but quite subdued,
Those early days seemed rough and rude.
As time went by I did recoup.
It dawned on me. I got the scoop.

I said it before and say it now.
Explain these things at time of vow.
I think I'm right, you're never wrong.
Descriptive words–unhappy song!

Now that I'm old and somewhat gray,
I've come to learn what I must say.
The key you ask and wait to hear.
My last words now, "Yes, dear! Yes, dear!"

---

105

Come by and visit some time…(I know that you're not going to come anyway).

---

# The Empty Nest

### I

A teardrop loudly splashed
Across the phone receiver.
'Twas not enough to disconnect
Or interrupt the hope.

That solitary drop
Was the flood
That  emptied
All the fertile chambers of my home and heart.

### II

Somewhere between parenthood
And grandparenthood
A vacuum cleaner appeared.
Indiscriminate! Deliberate!
Controlled by cold, malicious hands,
It challenged value by value, dream by dream,
And goal by goal in its path
Before I pulled the plug.

### III

Conceal
What's real.
Mask
The task.

Skirt around the core.
Supply hollow words galore
Multiplied more and more.
My heart is still sore.

I feel alone.
The pain cuts to the bone.
Send it to the Throne,
Whether bee or drone.

I wait for the best
Who passed the test.
I pause on the crest
Of my empty nest.

———————◆◆◆———————

**If you need anything please call... (those were just parting words–don't take me seriously).**

———————◆◆◆———————

# If My Pillow Could Talk

Rose patterns on my pillowcase kept vigil just like me.
They hid the teardrops from my face to mask my privacy.
The evidence of heartfelt payers ascended high to God.
Few people in my circle knew the lonely road I trod.

His pillows had rose petals, too, but hid no teardrop stain.
He seemed oblivious to price of daily heartfelt pain.
In jungle dense and modern town with tired feet I went.
Survival was my special gift though youthful substance spent.

My pillow does not judge his heart but looks at what he did.
His schemes caused us to drift apart his plans to leave he hid.
So now you know a little bit about the silent years.
The patterns on my pillowcase are really my own tears.

———————◆◆◆———————

**I was just thinking about you...(but don't ask me what I was thinking).**

# Saigon Pickpocket

Amidst the untamed traffic of bicycles, motor bikes, and people,
The Saigon thoroughfare bustled.
Above the din, a burst of laughter turned my head.
The sound came from twelve feet away, in front and to my right.
As if synchronized, I felt a touch from behind.
The noise distracted me from the touch of feathered fingers
That missed their mark. Confused,
I looked back, then to the front, and to the rear again.
Six eyes met.
We three laughed.
And disappeared in the swarming streets
With my wallet safely hidden elsewhere.

**The more ridiculous the reaction is to a seemingly simple matter, the deeper
is the significance of the behavior.**

# Sighs

Sighs.
Private sounds
Expelled
Without words.
Messages from the soul
Without explanation
But not devoid of meaning!

# Too Busy

Can't stay.
Don't want to be late.
Got too much on my plate.

Favorite verse? "Jesus Wept."
Longest name? Mahershalalhashbaz.
Settle for "Al" or just "Baz."

Can't talk.
No time to listen.
Might commit.

Eat on the run.
Disposable plate.
Take back-road.
Save time.

Access data.
High-speed modem.
Food cold.
Microwave too slow.

Quick glance.
Stop sign.
Take a chance.

Flesh competed
With metal!
And came in second.
Ambulance on time.

Coming to visit
Protégée?
Can't stay.
Out of the way.

Fast Burial Service Package,
Prerecorded program,
Crowded parlor schedule.
Wait your turn.
No viewing. No mourners.
Have time now.
Can't use it.

**You will pass on to your children what you brought from your heritage unless you make an effort to change it.**

# I Can't Get Through

Before I finish asking Dad
The question on my mind,
He steps right in as if he's mad
No time for me could find.

He's had a way with words, you know,
Since I was just a kid.
And when I try my love to show
I almost have to bid.

The topic does not matter much,
The outcome is the same.
I have to scheme to get a touch
And make of it a game.

Sometimes I'd say, "Just hear me out."
That wouldn't help a bit.
He's always right. Without a doubt
I'd end up in a fit.

My dad is an authority
On subjects, widely read.
But when the focus comes on me
I think the guy's brain dead.

I know he cares in other ways;
I think sometimes he tries.
He must have had some awful days–
I see it in his eyes.

Grandpa and Dad don't get along;
What hurtful history!
I want to sing a different song
Between my son and me.

# Lost Luggage

O Experience, great teacher, let me know what you will about loosing a piece of my luggage in the hotel lobby on my trip to a wedding in Jamaica. My precious conveniences: a pair of celestial binoculars, four banded neck dress shirts, a pair of black dress shoes that needed shining, my wife's portable hair dryer, her special Women's Bible with its carrying case – all gone; even my water pick whose regular use gave me the confidence to converse at close range so that people would not turn away from me politely with one hand partially covering their sensitive nostrils. All have unwillingly abandoned me for the shameful comfort of some modern day Mo Bay pirate.

"Yo room not ready. So go heat. Heat hall yo warnt. Yo luggage safe." My Seiko watch of sixteen years registered 2:25 pm. I trusted the fake welcome smile of the check-in clerk. He was a clean-cut local citizen trying to get ahead in the corporate world. I ate. I ate all I wanted in obedient response to the eager invitation showered upon me. I did not stop to remember the gradual threat of my love handles to join in front of me and obscure my fading abdominal muscles. I thought to myself, "I am loosing my youthful profile. Now I am loosing a piece of luggage too: the special one with the items I planned to wear to the wedding."

So my turn came! Three weeks earlier one of my cousins visited the USA from Trinidad. She lost her luggage in Atlanta and had to wear borrowed clothes to the wedding she came to attend. Oh that I could have learned the lost luggage lesson by proxy. The confident bellhops told me in rehearsed succession, "Yo left hit hat the hairport. Hit can't disappear from the lobby 'ere like dat. Na man." Likewise, I retorted, "I last saw all of my suitcases in your crowded hotel lobby when I regis-tered. Now one piece was missing." With each verbal cycle I make a desperate effort to keep down the loudness and pitch of my frustrated voice. Nevertheless, I began to feel the adrenaline surging through the pulsating arteries in my temples. Any observant bystander could have easily counted the pulse at my sweaty temples. Call it impatience! Call it intolerance for inefficiency! Call it unfinished business from my roller coaster past! You decide! Your answer would not return the lost items.

Then came silence from my supportive wife whose intended words of comfort unfortunately produced the opposite effect. My beloved helpmeet now bore the brunt of my displaced hostility. I paused and privately scrutinized the disappointing surroundings in disbelief after taking our other pieces of luggage ourselves to the safety of our room. To my detective eyes the spacious hotel lobby exhibited no sense of safety from the mishaps possible to unwary property. From my vantage point, the unattended luggage looked like penguins congregating with their backs turned on a shaded iceberg. At the same time, my Trinidadian mind pictured the frustrating scene as satisfied scavenging birds lined up on the outstretched branches of low-lying coconut trees awaiting their next meal.

With little room to spare between the ill-defined area for suitcases and seating for guests, swim suits and cargo pants sauntered back and forth at close range. The females appeared to cover as little of their modeled bodies as was legal, while their male counterparts camouflaged as much of their pseudo pregnant frames as the latest style displayed. This unscheduled vacationers' parade provided ample entertainment for my cautious eyes and sanctified imagination. Further slipper feet, sandal feet, high heel feet, flat heel feet, platform feet, sneaker feet, and bare feet all pitter-pattered pass me. I did not need free entertainment! I needed my conveniences! Who said that airport carousels, custom storage bays, hotel lobbies, hotel rooms, and thieves were incapable of concocting cruel jokes?

Then came the standoff. The bell captain and I tried to be gracious and civil, at least on the surface, without exceeding an unconscious international threshold for hostility. Laughter in the lobby repeatedly traded places with pulsating disco sounds from the poolside not too far away. A cool breeze whisked across our faces: a pleasant reminder that the quiet ocean still bathed the private beach that I purposefully ignored until then. Slurred speech and glazed eyes of the vacationers exposed the sultry effects of intoxication from lingering liquid stomach contents or saturated ganja lungs.

Between listening to reports of lack of progress toward the illusive goal, I shared my plight with captive listeners who ventured to sit nearby. I did not ask their reason for the pause or if they had the time to listen to me. I simply told them the story–the updated versions–that did not change except for the number of fruitless telephone calls the hotel staff said that they made to the airport and the increasing number of hotel rooms that were searched thus far. My troubled facial expression mirrored more of the electro-psycho-bio-chemical changes in my body than I intended to expose. Meanwhile, I tried to give the impression that I was relaxed, and my captive audience gave me pleasant nods, words of advice, fervent wishes for success, and promises of prayers. Prayers? Yes, prayers. They were not all infidels.

One guest even agreed to stop smoking where we sat. She willingly put out her cigarette but was a little miffed by my indirect approach. You see, I had asked her if she knew whether or not the hotel lobby was a "no-smoking area." "If you don't want me to smoke just say so." Her initially stern voice later relaxed as she added, "I don't need it anyway. I really don't mind. I just took some pain medication." That being said, she and her husb', I mean she and her male companion, who suddenly appeared, walked away. It is no wonder she was kind to me. We were fellow sufferers of sorts.

## Part II

Twenty-four hours after reaching for the Pullman that evaded my grasp in the hotel lobby I met with yet another employee for what the bellhop labeled an 'interview.' Finally, I thought, "I am about to have an official session that would bring relief for my loss." He interviewed me. He did not interrogate me. There is a difference! He put me at ease effortlessly. He condensed my (by now memorized) account on to one page with several blank spaces that did not apply. This gentleman of imposing size, pleasant voice, and mesmerizing mannerism avoided the computer on his desk. Instead he filled out the form longhand. I watched him closely. He did not even leave his desk to photocopy my list of traitor items. Instead, he called someone else to do it. By now I had begun to detach myself from my previously precious possessions. Still under his spell, I stood up when he did. He extended his giant right hand. I responded by reflex. "We will search the rooms of all the guests who arrived on the same day as you did, again, and get back with you." No, he did not drop any h's or apply them where they didn't belong. I thanked him profusely (for nothing). Still no luggage!

Sleep. Wake. Resume the front desk-lobby-management office vigil. More of the same! Well, time for a change.

The on-site attractions I ignored until now strangely beckoned me. Local artists peddled their works of art and reduced the listed prices before I could even make an offer. Watercraft sports pointed their inviting fingers at me and called out my name. An uneven water polo game struggled momentarily for my attention and lost it easily. Dark-skinned people cooled off in the shallow azure waters. Light-skinned people in search of a tropical tan lingered lazily in the blazing sun and had to settle immediately for the red burning version. What a price to pay for an exotic appearance! Leaning back on my blue fabric plastic-framed lounge chair in the cool shade of an almond tree, I raised my head long enough to follow an imaginary path in the water from the transparent shoreline twenty feet away out to the distinct horizon. What a gorgeous sight! In between those two points a kaleidoscope of shades of blue in the water responded obediently to the interplay of swiftly moving clouds and dancing rays of sunlight above. I wondered what the sunset would be like. No, I did not wait to find out.

Just then I realized that I had rediscovered relaxation, repose, and rest. For a few moments I did not need the luggage or even miss the contents. Big discovery! Life goes on! How interesting! Those were the very words I uttered to myself three weeks earlier when my cousin lost her luggage. I could not tell her that out loud. We would have resumed our lifelong mutual badgering contest.

## Part III

And now for the resolution–actually the beginning of the resolution! At my second meeting with the "gentle giant," I tried to take charge of the session. At an opportune moment I persuaded him to give me a copy of his report that I had expected to be named Lost and Found. Diplomatically it was called the Guest Incident Report Form. How soothing! He promptly volunteered me to take the original to a young lady in another section of the wood and glass maze. I knew then that I had lost control of the undeclared contest. When I arrived at her section I recognized her immediately. She was the assistant manager to whom I had privately protested at the check-in counter one day earlier after the bride whose wedding I came to attend called her to intervene on my behalf.

Something dawned on me at that moment: I came to understand the basis for selecting successful employees in tourism or public relations. This lady's charming smile disarmed me and eased the severity of my inconvenience. She really did not have to say much. Actually she could not do much either. My luggage played hide and seek while I, a former member of the American College of Physician Executives, functioned as a conscripted errand boy arranging for my own documents. What a vacation! I left her desk-littered office with a copy of the Guest Incident Report Form but not before I insisted on getting the name and address of the hotel's insurance adjuster. Of course, she couldn't locate their business cards or letterhead stationery on her desk. She had to go to another office to get the information. As she handed me a piece of paper three inches square she said softly, "You will hear from us in about two weeks." This was my consoling dismissal. I placed the yellow sticky on my prized piece of paper that now represented the lost luggage, and we parted pleasantly. My frustration tried to erupt. It could not. The piece of paper soothed my fragile nerves. I finally had concrete evidence of my loss.


## Part IV

Now I had to prepare myself for two weeks of waiting for a response from the insurance adjuster. This time would no doubt amount to reviewing each step covered thus far with the usual double-checking of the answers–again. After all, the suitcase of one of their clients just could not disappear from the lobby of the busy resort hotel. After all, other tourists had thought they saw their luggage at the hotel when it had been misplaced at the airport or in transit elsewhere. After all, other hotel guests had casually ignored abandoned luggage in their room because it was not bothering them.

Wait for two weeks! On to Trinidad! I wondered what time measurement standard to use: the businessperson's can't-loose-a-minute clock; the "It's-not-our-fault" stalling technique of the hotel staff; or the casual "no-rush" pace of a developing country's culture? Perhaps during this period I would learn how to wait without being idle. I waited. I enjoy the rest of my vacation while learning how to adjust without my conveniences.

But I have not told you the whole account. Where was my toilet article bag? Where was our emergency snack just in case the airline did not feed us? Where was a change of shirt and pajamas that might come in handy? Where were my two Bibles, one with the large print and all marked up, the other small and compact? Where was my Sabbath School Bible Study Guide? Where were my sermon materials? Where was my poetry notebook with all kinds of ideas at different stages of completion? It is no small wonder that my carry-on bag was so heavy. Fortunately, that piece was not stolen. My wife had cast a sympathetic eye in my direction at regular intervals even before my terrible loss. She had seen my aging frame struggle without verbal complaint. Now it was worse. We transferred our own luggage and deprived the porters of their ever-present tip. You know what I mean: tip from car to sidewalk check-in counter; tip from baggage claim to customs; tip to shuttle bus; tip to hotel lobby; tip to storage; tip to hotel room. Now that's a legal racket if I ever saw one! I suppose these porters report their annual income truthfully at income tax filing time! Yes, for real! Besides, they were not going to get an opportunity to steal another piece of our suitcases or carry on luggage.

My wife was particularly careful not to say out loud what she was thinking. In order to compensate for the heaviness of the carry-on bag and pull two pieces of rolling suitcases, I leaned to one side. I just knew she was thinking that I looked like a donkey cart rolling along with one wheel larger than the other or a vehicle with flat tires on one side. After 39 years of marriage you get to know these things. She did not have to speak. In fact, she dared not. Prior experience taught her that under certain conditions the male hormone testosterone converts into venom, and Bible-toting heaven-bound husbands transform into spitting cobras with poor aim. Heaven bound? Where is the nearest baptistery? But for all it's worth, the useful contents of the carry-on bag compensated for the extra weight. I was grateful that it did not abandon me also. I became philosophical and mused privately, "Success frequently results from temporary inconveniences."


## Part V

Now let's take a look at some lessons I learned from loosing my luggage. First, some lessons have to be learned by experience, not by proxy. Second, life has to go on in spite of the loss of priceless possessions. Third, if I want a successful outcome, I must be prepared for some temporary inconveniences. Fourth, it occurred to me that there were several kinds of waiting: 1) Patient waiting, like accepting any outcome; 2) Unhappy waiting, like worrying about all of the "what ifs;" 3)

Prepared waiting, like following the instructions given during the interim; 4) Unprepared waiting, like leaving the results to chance; 5) Lying in wait to do harm and take revenge. I am sure there are others.

All of us have lost something at one time or another. Behavioral experts agree that how you deal with trauma may be more important than what actually happened, as devastating as that might be. What losses have you suffered a long time ago or recently: job, money, friend, opportunity, spouse, parent, child, priceless possession, and something that was insignificant to others but precious to you? The list can go on. How are you dealing with the loss?

Adam and Eve lost our luggage in the Garden of Eden a long time ago, and we are feeling the effects to this day. They lost innocence. They lost face-to-face communication with God. They lost protection from evil and its fatal results. They lost a lot more, and we are still waiting for the full replacement. Grace, mercy, forgiveness, unconditional love, tolerance, and hope soothe our mortal aches and pains. Meanwhile, we suffer and wait. We wait and suffer. The extent to which we submit our lives to Jesus, the Great Luggage Locater and Replacer, determines how we cope in this life and where we will spend eternity.

As it was in the case of my surgical ordeal, the personal and spiritual lessons I learned from losing my luggage were opportunities to let the Lord have His way in my life. For the rest of my trip I substituted items as needed or purchased others where necessary. I lost a piece of luggage and learned some valuable lessons in exchange. The lost luggage claim process continued unsuccessfully for over four months at the last count. Upon my return to Atlanta none of the three pieces of our remaining baggage arrived with our plane. All we had was our carry-on pieces. But that's another story.

# AFTERWORD

The past two years of my life have been a time of healing of body, mind, and spirit. I am grateful to God and all of my supporters for their guidance and assistance. I glory in the lessons I learned from my experiences. Indeed, GOD'S GRACE IS SUFFICIENT FOR ME **(G.G.I.S.F.M.)**.

If some item in this collection helps someone to cope with any challenge of life not necessarily related to prostate cancer; if it adds a deeper, spiritual dimension to a worship service; if it prompts a reader to take health checks more seriously; then I would consider this book to be a success. In this enlightened age, men at risk for developing prostate cancer do not have to die from the illness. Get help, early!

On September 11, 2016. On a flight #   e from Detroit to Atlanta GA I had a fortune to met this wonderful human being. mr. Rudy Broomers. I was standing on the side were passanger were standing ready to aboard the Plane when I saw mr. Rudy walk by. then he aboard first then few minutes later me, then what a surpris: he was on the same raw sit. right next to me. e first he was very quite. playing crosswords on his cell phone, I was reading[117] a booor.

"maximum Achievement" by brian tracy.
(maxima eficacia). then after being reading
for a 30minutes. I deeide to take a nap
of 15minutes. then I was curious to turn
am my head and I asked mr. Rudy if he was
a prastor or priest and he look at me and
smile.

Copies of

# SUFFICIENT GRACE:
### SURVIVING PROSTATE CANCER

May be ordered from:

**Rudlauv Publishers**
P.O. Box 70893
Tuscaloosa, AL 35407-0893

Name _____

Address _____

_____

City _____ State _____ Zip _____


_____ Copies @    US  $ 19.95  per copy  $ _____

Alabama residents add    US  $ 1.80  per copy  $ _____

Shipping and handling    US  $ 3.00          $ _____

Total Enclosed                                $ _____